Engineering Hemodynamics: Application to Cardiac Assist Devices

Engineering Hemodynamics: Application to Cardiac Assist Devices

Walter Welkowitz
Rutgers University

Lexington Books
D.C. Heath and Company
Lexington, Massachusetts
Toronto

Library of Congress Cataloging in Publication Data

Welkowitz, Walter, 1926–
Engineering hemodynamics.
Includes bibliographical references and index.
1. Hemodynamics—Mathematical models. 2. Biomedical engineering. 3. Pacemaker, Artificial (Heart) I. Title. [DNLM: 1. Assisted circulation. 2. Heart, Mechanical. 3. Hemodynamics. WG168 W446e]
QP105.W46 599'.01'1 76-53921
ISBN 0-669-01300-5

Published simultaneously in Canada

Printed in the United States of America

International Standard Book Number: 0-669-01300-5

Library of Congress Catalog Card Number: 76-53921

To Joan, David, Larry, and Julie

Contents

List of Figures

List of Tables

List of Symbols

a	major semiaxis of eipsoidal ventricle model
b	minor semiaxis of ellipsoidal ventricle model
c_j	circular cylinder subdivision of left ventricle
e	magnitude error between model and measured pressure transfer functions
e_θ	phase error between model and measured pressure transfer functions
f	frequency
f^k	transitional functional relationship
g_i	model pressure transfer function in aorta, ith frequency
h_a	aorta wall thickness
h_v	ventricle wall thickness
h_{v1}	ventricle wall thickness of unimpaired segment
h_{v2}	ventricle wall thickness of impaired segment
k	taper coefficient of aorta
l	length of aorta section
l_1	length of unimpaired segment of ventricle
l_2	length of impaired segment of ventricle
l_{11}	length of unimpaired segment of ventricle at end diastole
l_{12}	length of impaired segment of ventricle at end diastole
$p(t)$	left ventricule pressure during systole
r_a	radius of aorta
r_{a2}	radius of aorta at femoral bifurcation
r_v	radial coordinate of left ventricle
r_{vj}	radius of jth segment of ventricle model
r_{v1j}	radius of jth segment of ventricle at end diastole
s	complex frequency ($j\omega$ for steady-state excitation)
t_{pi}	measured pressure transfer function in aorta, ith frequency

$u(k)$	pump control variables
w	weighting factor
x	coordinate of ellipsoidal ventricle
y	coordinate of ellipsoidal ventricle
z	longitudinal coordinate
A	area
A_a	cross-sectional area of aorta
A_{a0}	aorta cross-sectional area at diastole
A_{av}	average cross-sectional area of length of aorta
A_h	cross-sectional area of cylindrical wall
A_T	transmission coefficient for aorta section
A_v	ventricle cross-sectional area
A_z	complex impedance function
B_T	transmission coefficient for aorta section
B_z	complex impedance function
C	hydraulic capacitance
C_a	hydraulic capacitance of aortic section per unit length
C_{a1}	hydraulic capacitance per unit length at aortic input
C_{a2}	hydraulic capacitance per unit length at bifurcatton
C_{ai}	hydraulic series capacitance-input to aorta
C_f	hydraulic capacitance of section of femoral artery
C_{pj}	parallel capacitance of circuit model of left ventricle, *j*th segment
C_T	transmission coefficient for aorta section
C_v	elastic constant in segmental ventricle model
C_z	complex impedance function
D_T	transmission coefficient for aorta section
D_z	complex impedance function
E	Young's modulus of elasticity
E_{a2}	modulus of elasticity of aorta wall at bifurcation

E_p	elastic coefficient $\left(\frac{\Delta p}{\Delta r_a} \cdot r_a\right)$
E_{v1}	elasticity of unimpaired ventricle wall at end diastole
E_{v2}	elasticity of impaired ventrical wall at end diastole
E'_{v2}	elasticity of impaired ventricle wall during systole
F	force
F_θ	circumferential force in a cylindrical segment
$G_j(t)$	an isometric force $(\pi r_{vj}(t)T_s)$
H^k	Hamiltonian function
J	performance index
J_1	performance index
J_2	performance index
K_v	viscosity parameter $(8\pi\nu/A_v)$
L	heart muscle segment length (can be circumference)
L_a	inertance of blood in section of aorta
L_{ai}	hydraulic series inertance-aorta input
L_{a0}	average inertance parameter $(\rho l_a/A_{\text{av}})$
L_f	hydraulic inertance of section of femoral artery
L_{sj}	series inductance of circuit model of left ventricle jth segment
L^k	a function
N	number of circular cylinders into which ventricle is subdivided
P	presure
P_a	aortic pressure
P_f	pressure at ideal flow source operating alone
P_g	equivalent source pressure
P_0	end diastolic pressure
P_s	mean equivalent source pressure
P_v	left ventricular pressure
P_1	aortic root pressure
P'_1	mean aortic root pressure during assisted circulation

P_{11}	aortic root pressure without pumping
P_{12}	aortic root pressure with pump alone, no heart source
P_2	aortic pressure proximal to femoral bifurcation
P_{2m}	phasor component of P_2
Q	volumetric flow
Q_a	aortic flow
Q_f	ideal source flow
Q'_f	average ideal source flow
Q_m	figure of merit $(f_r/\Delta f)$
Q_s	zero-load flow
Q_1	aortic root flow
Q'_1	mean aortic root flow during assisted circulation
Q_{11}	aortic root flow without pumping
Q_{12}	aortic root flow with pump alone, no heart source
Q_2	aortic flow proximal to femoral bifurcation
Q_{2m}	phasor component of Q_2
R_a	hydraulic resistance of aorta section per unit length
R_{a1}	hydraulic resistance of aorta section per unit length at aortic input
R_{a2}	hydraulic resistance of aortic section per unit length, proximal to femoral bifurcation
R_{ai}	hydraulic series input resistance of aorta
R_{aT}	hydraulic series resistance of aorta termination
R_f	hydraulic resistance of section of femoral artery
R_i	inside radius of aorta at any point
R_{pj}	parallel resistance of circuit model of left ventricle, jth segment
R_s	equivalent ventricle source internal resistance
R_{sj}	series resistance of circuit model of left ventricle, jth segment
R_T	terminal resistance
R_v	aortic valve hydraulic resistance

R_x	series resistance of aorta section between assist pump and femoral bifurcation
R_1, R_2	radii of curvature of ellipsoid model of ventricle
T	tension ($F/\Delta z$ in a cylindrical section of left ventricle)
T_m	matrix transpose
T_P	pressure transfer function
T_Q	flow transfer function
T_θ	circumferential tension in a cylindrical segment
T_s	isometric tension in an active ventricle strip
V_a	cylindrical approximation to volume of ellipsoidal model of ventricle
V_m	ventricle muscle wall velocity
V_0	end diastolic volume of left ventricle
V_v	volume of ellipsoidal model of ventricle
V_{max}	maximum ventricle muscle wall velocity
W_a	aortic hydraulic power
W_g	hydraulic equivalent source power
W_v	ventricular hydraulic power
$X(k)$	state variables of pumped circulatory system
XFi	desired aortic hemodynamic condition
Y	error measure
Z_a	aortic hydraulic impedance
Z_g	equivalent ventricle source internal impedance
Z_T	terminal impedance
Z_v	aortic valve hydraulic impedance
Z_0	characteristic impedance of aortic section
Z_1	hydraulic impedance at aortic root (input impedance)
$\hat{Z}_1$	aortic input impedance, lumped circuit model of aorta
Z_{11}	aortic input impedance, without pumping
Z_2	aortic impedance proximal to femoral bifurcation (terminating impedance)

Z_{2m}	frequency component of $Z_2(P_{2m}/Q_{2m})$
β	bulk modulus of blood
β_e	hoop elasticity
γ	$(k^2 + sR_{a2}C_{a2})^{1/2}$
θ	phase angle
θ_g	phase angle of fundamental component of source pressure
θ_j	angular dimension of impaired cylindrical section
$\theta(z)$	angular dimension of impaired section as a function of longitudinal coordinate
$\lambda(k)$	Lagrangian multiplier
ν	blood viscosity
ν_{eff}	"effective" blood viscosity
π	3.141 . . .
ρ	blood density
ρ_0	average blood densiiy
ρ_r	reflection coefficient
σ	active stress of heart muscle segment
σ_a	average circumferential stress over left ventricle
σ_s	isometric stress of heart muscle segment
σ_{R1}, σ_{R2}	longitudinal and circumferential stresses in heart wall at radii of curvature locations R_1 and R_2
σ_{av}	spatially averaged maximum isovolumic wall stress for left ventricle
σ_1	stress in unimpaired heart muscle segment
σ_2	stress in impaired heart muscle segment
ω	angular frequency
Δ	a small change
ϕ	a function

Foreword

Engineering Hemodynamics: Application to Cardiac Assist Devices treats the dynamics of the living circulatory system through the use of analytical techniques used extensively by electrical engineers. This book is part of a series being developed by the Lexington Books Division of D.C. Heath and Company on subjects of current interest to electrical engineers.

Few persons question the goal of attacking the world's medical problems by applying the combined techniques and knowledge of the medical and technical communities. However, the difficulties of communications between disciplines continue to impede progress because almost every problem requires the combined talents of the physician, the life scientist, the physical scientist, and the engineer. This book contains an important body of knowledge obtained from an extensive research effort that has applied modern engineering analysis techniques to living systems. A hint at the communications problems involved in the bioengineering field is given by a sampling of words from the book: ventricle, vascular system, ellipsoidal shell model, source impedance, nonuniform hybrid model, isovolumic stress, complex frequency, matrix transpose, state variables, Lagrangian multiplier.

This book considers the circulatory system by first describing the mechanical features of major anatomical parts in mathematical terms. Then, equivalent electrical networks are developed for the left ventricle, the aortic valve, the aorta, and the peripheral circulatory system. In order to obtain simple and yet meaningful mathematical models, it was necessary to conduct an extensive experiment program. The book includes physiological justifications for the various mathematical simplifications used. Studies of the overall circulatory system also are discussed. To investigate the overall system, it is structured analytically as a complex electrical network comprised of the individual equivalent circuits used for each major anatomical function. Effects of mechanical interactions generated by heart assist devices are analyzed by using the complex network to determine overall effects on the circulatory system. Considerable attention is given in the book to the use of these analyses for improving the performance of automatic controls for living systems. Other applications of the analyses that have also proved useful are discussed in the last chapter.

Maurice W. Long

Preface

Over a span of about ten years the biomedical engineering group in the department of electrical engineering of Rutgers University has been carrying out a program of analysis of the various physiological characteristics of the systemic circulatory system. The anatomical segments studied included the aorta, the aortic valve, the left ventricle, the peripheral arterial system, and the nerve controls to the heart. In addition system analysis procedures were applied to the problems of mechanically assisted circulation.

This book incorporates these various separate studies into a comprehensive hemodynamic analysis of the systemic circulation. This analysis includes the formulation of physical equations describing the functions of the hemodynamic entities and the integration of the isolated descriptions into an overall system with discussions of overall performance.

The various isolated studies represent the efforts of many members of the biomedical engineering group and the author would like to take this opportunity to thank his colleagues and students—Professors Sylvan Fich, Donald Molony, Byoung Min, and Drs. Joseph Strano, Shirish Shastri, Robert Watts—for their contributions to this work. In addition the surgical research group at Sinai Hospital in Detroit—Dr. Adrian Kantrowitz, Dr. Dov Jaron, and Mr. Paul Freed—deserve much thanks for the experimental verification studies related to this work. Finally, I am indebted to Mrs. Constance Zylman for typing the manuscript and to many publishers and authors who gave me permission to repoduce figures from the literature. These include the Alliance for Engineering in Medicine and Biology for material appearing in the Annual Conferences on Engineering in Medicine and Biology; the New York Academy of Sciences for material appearing in the Transactions of the New York Academy of Sciences; the IEEE for material appearing in the Transactions on Biomedical Engineering; the Instrument Society of America for material appearing in the Proceedings of the 7th Rocky Mountain Symposium; and the Bulletin of Mathematical Biology for material appearing in that journal.

In addition, S. Karger, AG Basel granted permission to reproduce Figures 5–5 through 5–12 from *Bibliotheca Cardiologica*, 29, pp. 14–27 (1972). Pergamon Press, Inc. granted permission to reproduce Figures 2–1 through 2–5 from *International Journal of Engineering Science*, 11, pp. 601–611 (© 1973) and Figures 3–25, 3–26 from *International Journal of Engineering Science*, 10, pp. 1081–1091 (© 1972). Edward Arnold Ltd.

granted permission to reproduce Figure 3–7 from D. A. McDonald, *Blood Flow in Arteries*. Figures 5–1 through 5–4 were originally presented at the 143rd Spring Meeting of the Electrochemical Society, Inc. in Chicago, Ill. and are included in the publication *Proceedings of Electrochemical Bioscience Symposium* of the Electrochemical Society, Inc.

Engineering Hemodynamics: Application to Cardiac Assist Devices

1 Introduction

Physiology is historically a descriptive and experimental science. However, certain anatomical systems such as the circulatory system are mainly mechanical in nature and lend themselves to the same mathematical physics analysis so common in the study of mechanics and hydrodynamics. While we tend to think of mathematical biology as a very recent field, the applications of mathematical physics to the study of bood flow go back to the time of Euler in the eighteenth century and continue through the early nineteenth century with the work of Young and the middle of that century with the efforts of the Weber brothers (Noordergraaf 1969). Since that time the activities directed toward the mathematical analysis of hemodynamics have been very extensive and often reviewed (Noordergraaf 1969; Talbot and Gessner 1973; Cope 1965). In order to contribute to this extensively studied field, an attempt has been made to apply modern electrical engineering techniques to the investigation of the hemodynamics of the systemic circulation. These techniques include the methods of nonuniform transmission line analysis, the use of hybrid lumped distributed networks, impedance function and transfer function analysis, control system parameter identification procedures, synthesis of equivalent networks, and applications of computer simulation programs to the analysis of large-scale multimesh networks.

While the work described in this book is heavily analytical, it has been continuously accompanied by extensive experimental studies, primarily on dogs. This experimental phase has been most vital, since mathematical procedures in physiology require simplified models which can easily be in error and therefore must be continuously verified experimentally.

The anatomical portions of the circulatory system that are discussed include the left ventricle, the aortic valve, the aorta, the peripheral arterial system, and the neural controls to the heart. System analysis is applied to the problems of mechanically assisted circulation, diagnosis of disorders of the major vessels, and diagnosis of left ventricular myocardial infarction. The approach taken in this book includes the formulation of physical equations describing the functions of the hemodynamic entities and the integration of isolated descriptions into an overall system description. The performance of this overall system during assisted circulation is extensively described. Inherent in the analyses presented are simplifications which make the equations mathematically tractable. Also included are the physiological justifications for these simplifications. It is expected that the results of this engineering analysis of the systemic circulation will contribute to the overall physiological understanding of blood flow.

Three chapters in this book are devoted to three specific anatomical entities—the left ventricle, the aorta, and the peripheral systemic circulation. The remaining chapters present a systems approach to assisted circulation. The engineering techniques used to elucidate the physiological functions depend upon the anatomical application.

1.1 Left Ventricle

A number of techniques are presented with respect to the performance of the left ventricle. Some detailed muscle models are explored and analytically related to ventricular contraction. An equivalent source network representation is developed, and an experimental technique for measuring it is discussed. An ellipsoidal hollow shell model is explored, and its properties are related both to the equivalent source network and to muscle models. In this manner, indices for evaluating left ventricular performance are developed. Finally, an ellipsoidal shell model with an arbitrary defective region (infarct) is analyzed, and a network equivalent for this system is evolved. Predictions from these different models are compared with measurements obtained on dogs with induced heart failure.

1.2 Aorta

The hemodynamic relationship between pressure and the flow of blood in the aorta is elucidated by considering fluid mechanical equations for a fluid-filled thin-walled tapered tube of nonuniform properties. The emphasis in the solutions presented is on the effects of the geometric tapering and the elastic nonuniformities. Approximate solutions are obtained for the complex sets of equations by using methods taken from nonuniform transmission line analysis. By using a parameter identification and optimization procedure, in conjunction with the mathematical models of the aorta and pressure measurements within the aorta, calculations of the physical properties of the aorta such as diameter, taper, and wall elasticity are presented. This technique for the identification of aorta parameters appears to be applicable to the diagnosis of arterial diseases.

1.3 Peripheral Vascular System

Various analytical and experimental techniques are described for examining the reflection of blood pressure waves from the peripheral vascular system back toward the heart. Calculations demonstrate that the amount of wave energy reflected is very small and that the transmission system is well matched—almost all the pulsatile wave energy is outgoing.

A number of network models are presented in an attempt to explain the performance of peripheral blood vessels under dilation and constriction. Drug experiments which attempt to validate the network models are discussed.

1.4 Analysis of Assisted Circulation

The individual models are joined into an overall model of systemic circulation. By applying network superposition theorems, performance characteristics of mechanical heart assist devices are explored. Some conditions for optimum timing adjustment of assist devices are developed. Finally, a procedure is presented for computer control of pumping which readjusts the device as the myocardium is improved and determines when assistance can be terminated.

The material that appears in this book is a synthesis of approximately twenty individual studies that have been carried out since 1966. Appropriate references to individual studies are presented where applicable in each chapter.

References

Cope, F.W., "Elastic Reservoir Theories of the Human Circulation with Applications to Clinical Medicine and to Computer Analysis of the Circulation," in *Advances in Biological and Medical Physics* (New York: Academic Press, 1965), pp. 277–356.

Noordergraaf, A., "Hemodynamics," in H.P. Schwan, *Biological Engineering* (New York, McGraw-Hill, 1969).

Talbot, S.A., and Gessner, U., *Systems Physiology* (New York: Wiley-Interscience, 1973).

2 Analytical Dynamics of the Left Ventricle

Both from the point of view of understanding the detailed functioning of the heart and in using this understanding to diagnose problems of impaired hearts, an analytical representation of the functioning of the normal and the impaired left ventricle is quite useful. Such a representation will, of necessity, interrelate the mechanical properties of the ventricle wall with the hydrodynamic characteristics of the pumped blood. In this manner it can provide a rational basis for many of the indices that have been proposed and used to determine cardiac status. The search for simply measured hemodynamic indices that would describe the contractile state of the myocardium has been extensive, but many problems have been encountered in their use (Van Den Bos et al. 1973). Among the indices that have been studied are the maximum rate of rise of left ventricular pressure ($LV\,dP/dt$ max), the maximum rate of rise of left ventricular pressure divided by the left ventricular pressure at that time [($LV\,dP/dt$ max)/P], the maximum of the ratio of rate of rise to left ventricular pressure [($LV\,dP/dt/P$)max], and plots of some of these quantities against each other. It was found that these indices were sensitive to load and heart size under all circumstances (Van Den Bos et al. 1973) and, therefore, of little use in directly characterizing the state of the myocardium. Katz and Brady (1971) indicate that some direct muscle mechanical parameters such as maximum shortening velocity have both basic biophysical and basic biochemical dependencies and, therefore, would be more useful in determining cardiac state. Obviously, an analytical relationship between the hemodynamic parameters and the muscle mechanical parameters would greatly aid in the formulation of useful hemodynamic indices. As suggested, the size of the left ventricle varies in accordance with the Frank-Starling mechanism, and this variation limits the utility of many of the contractility indices. Thus a theoretical relationship between ventricle size and the hemodynamic parameters also would be most useful. Many diseases of the heart are due to localized disturbances (infarcts), which are produced by local blockages of the blood supply to the heart muscle. A successful analysis of ventricular performance must be able to take into account localized defects and relate these to average hemodynamic performance.

There is a variety of desirable information that an analysis of left ventricular performance can supply (Noordergraaf and Meester 1973;

Talbot 1973). Probably the most useful would be a method for computing the ability of the left ventricle to do the work necessary to pump blood around the systemic circulation. The power that the heart supplies in humans varies from about 2 to 10 W, depending upon exertion. The cardiac output varies from about 4 l/min at rest to about 15 l/min in strenuous exercise (Talbot and Gessner 1973). Thus for full performance, the heart must be capable of handling about 15 l/min of flow and generating about 10 W of hydrodynamic power. In addition to the ability of the left ventricle to perform work, its stability under sudden, large load changes is important. It has been observed that under appropriate physiological control, even an impaired heart can generate a normal cardiac output. However, under a sudden load change the controlled system may become unstable and no longer be able to carry the load.

If at all possible, an analytical exposition should permit calculation of the properties of the system from easily measurable quantities. These should be external measurements when feasible, so that the analytical methods can be applied to a variety of patients. Finally, analytical techniques should provide sufficiently detailed information so that they can be an aid in suggesting treatment in cases of impaired hearts.

The analysis presented in this chapter was developed at Rutgers University over a period of about six years. Portions of this work were incoporated in the doctoral theses of Shastri (1969), Min (1972), and Watts (1974).

A number of modeling techniques using both equivalent networks and mechanical shells are employed to interrelate the hemodynamic measurements with the muscle properties. The most basic strategy used is to simulate the left ventricle as an equivalent pressure source (Fich et al. 1973). In this approach, the left ventricle is considered as a pressure generator with a series impedance. Both of these are pulsatile, time-varying quantities. Their parameters can be evaluated approximately by applying two conditions of loading to the heart (Shastri 1969). One experimental procedure requires making measurements for both an unassisted heart and an assisted heart. An intra-aortic balloon pump can be used to provide the varied load conditions for this procedure. Partial cross clamping of the aorta has also been used to provide appropriate load variations.

In the presentation that follows dynamic shell models of the left ventricle are employed to interrelate the hemodynamic parameters with the equivalent pressure-source parameters. The properties of the shell walls are characterized by a variety of muscle models such as those of Hill (1938) and Carlson (1957). As suggested by Rushmer (1961), these shell models inherently assume circumferential muscle fibers lying in parallel planes.

These hypothetical fibers contribute most of the force needed for blood ejection.

Both thin-walled (Sandler and Dodge 1963) and thick-walled (Talbot and Gessner 1973) shell models have been analyzed. Hood et al. (1969) have shown that the mean stress as estimated from thin-wall models is close in value to that obtained using thick-wall models. The average stress obtained from thin-wall models is in good agreement with the mid-wall stress of the other models. Furthermore, Eggleton et al. (1970) have shown that during contraction there is extensive in-folding of the inner portion of the myocardium. The active stress-containing section of the myocardial wall actually may be fairly thin and well represented by a thin-wall model. In addition, since all the models used are only approximations to left ventricular geometry, there appears to be ample justification for using the simpler thin-wall rather than the complex and nonlinear thick-wall model.

A typical semiellipsoidal shell model of the left ventricle can be used only to represent average impaired properties of a defective heart. However, Watts (1974) found that by representing the ventricle as a plurality of thin-wall cylindrical shells, it is possible to take into account local properties (such as localized infarcts) and incorporate them into a model in terms of their geometries. Furthermore, by employing a force-voltage analog for each cylindrical section, it is possible to represent the entire left ventricle as a multimesh network. The circuit element values in the network represent physical parameters such as ventricular geometry, blood mass, and muscle tissue viscosity, elasticity, and contractile characteristics. The entire equivalent network can be readily exercised using digital computer network simulation programs, and the hydrodynamic characteristics of the system under various impairments can be studied.

By using the approaches mentioned, it has been possible to derive the following parameters that are most useful in studying the dynamics of the left ventricle:

1. equivalent source parameters (pressure and impedance) both as phasor quantities and as time-varying functions
2. average wall stress as a function of time in the cardiac cycle
3. left ventricular volume as a function of time in the cardiac cycle
4. a plot of stress versus volume as often used to present the Frank-Starling characteristics (this is obtainable by combining items 2 and 3)
5. isovolumic tension in the muscle wall
6. maximum muscle-shortening velocity
7. left ventricular shape and volume as a function of localized impairment
8. various pressure-volume relationships as a function of impairment

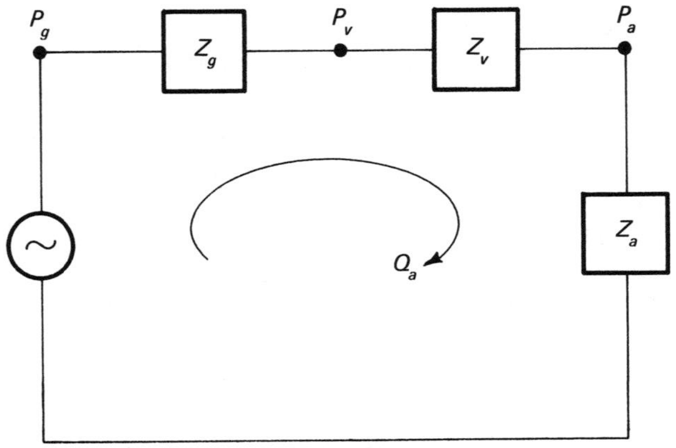

Figure 2–1 Equivalent Source Representation of the Heart.

2.1 Equivalent Source Representation

One technique that has been used to describe the left ventricle pumping blood into the systemic circulatory system is to model it as a pressure source in series with an hydraulic internal impedance. This approach lumps all the spatially distributed characteristics and all the diverse physical entities such as contractile strength, elasticity, and size into the Thevenin source equivalent. Such an approach is not unique in modeling but in fact is the most common approach used in describing electrical generators in analyzing electrical systems. By using this approach, a simplified lumped network representation of the systemic circulation is shown in Figure 2–1. In this figure P_g, P_v, and P_a correspond to the source pressure, left ventricular pressure, and aortic pressure, respectively. Z_g, Z_v, and Z_a correspond to the source impedance, valve impedance, and aortic impedance, respectively. The description used has been proposed by Shastri (1969) and Fich et al. (1973).

The six parameters illustrated in the figure are generally time-varying functions. When this time variation is of a steady-state pulsatile nature, Min (1972) has shown that the network of Figure 2–1 can be treated like a linear network with the quantities P_g, P_v, P_a, and Q_a (the aortic flow) resolvable into their Fourier components and representable by phasors. If we use these phasors, then at each frequency

$$Z_g = \frac{P_g - P_v}{Q_a} \tag{2–1}$$

$$Z_v = \frac{P_v - P_a}{Q_a} \tag{2–2}$$

$$Z_a = \frac{P_a}{Q_a} \tag{2–3}$$

Equation (2–1) can be rewritten as

$$P_g = P_v + Z_g \cdot Q_a \tag{2–4}$$

for each frequency.

The source phasor parameters P_g and Z_g are functions of the various physiological and mechanical properties of the heart. Determination of these phasor quantities can be carried out by utilizing two different load impedances (Z_a) and measuring the ventricular pressure and aortic flow for the two loads. It is assumed that the source parameters remain constant during the two measurements. By using subscripts 1 and 2 for the two loading conditions and applying phasor Eq. (2–4), the source pressure and impedance phasors are obtained from the relationships

$$P_g = \frac{P_{v1} \cdot Q_{a2} - P_{v2} \cdot Q_{a1}}{Q_{a2} - Q_{a1}} \tag{2–5}$$

and

$$Z_g = \frac{P_g - P_{v1}}{Q_{a1}} = \frac{P_g - P_{v2}}{Q_{a2}} \tag{2–6}$$

Rapid variation of the load on the heart can be carried out by utilizing an intra-aortic balloon pump. Two successive waveform complexes (with and without balloon pumping) can be used for the Fourier analysis calculations. An example of such measurements is shown in Figure 2–2. These measurements were made on a dog for the cases of a normal heart and a heart with induced failure. The requirement of constancy for P_g and Z_g under the load variation can be approximated by using successive waveform complexes, since Puri and Gido (1968) have estimated that the time constants of the cardiac control mechanisms are greater than a few seconds.

A typical discrete frequency spectrum of source pressure phasors as calculated using both Eq. (2–5) and measurements made on a dog before and after induced heart failure is shown in Figure 2–3. The corresponding source impedances as a function of frequency are shown in Figure 2–4. By using the pressure phasor components it is possible to reconstruct an equivalent pressure-source time function. A typical set of functions before and after induced heart failure as measured on a dog is shown in Figure 2–5. An examination of Figures 2–3, 2–4, and 2–5 shows that the magnitudes of the source parameters are quite sensitive to induced heart failure and in themselves may be useful parameters to characterize the heart. They are also useful as intermediate steps in determining other parameters.

2.2 Ellipsoidal Shell Model

The left ventricle is approximately egg-shaped. Rushmer (1961) has described the left ventricular cavity as a cylinder with a conoid segment at the apical end. A number of investigators (Koushanpour and Collings 1966; Vayo 1966) have modeled the left ventricle as a truncated ellipsoid of

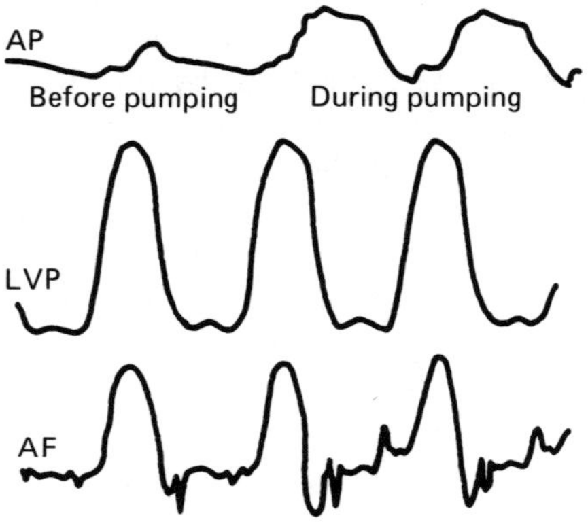

(*a*) Time domain variation of left ventricular pressure, LVP, aortic pressure, AP, and aortic flow, AF, in dog without induced failure, before and during pumping

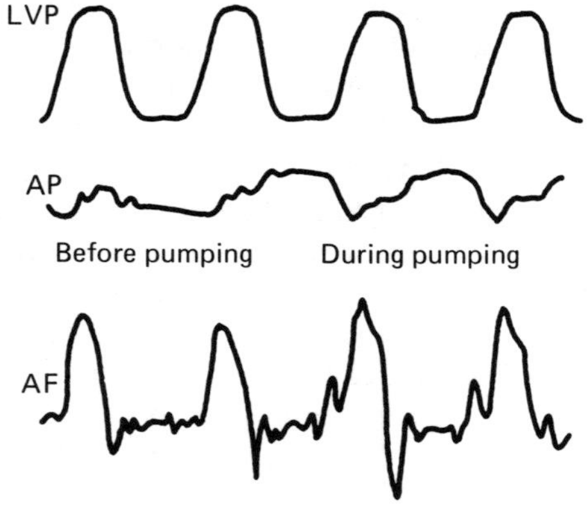

(*b*) Time domain variation of left ventricular pressure, LVP, aortic pressure, AP, and aortic flow, AF, in dog with induced failure, before and during pumping.

Figure 2–2 Loading Produced by Use of Intra-aortic Balloon Pump.

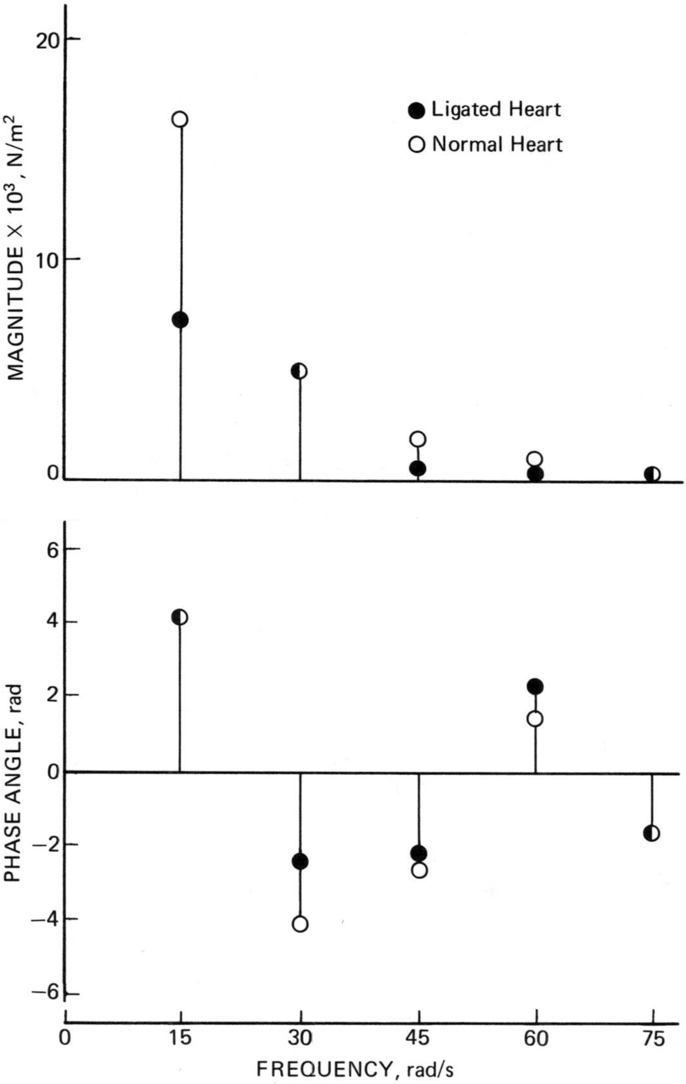

Figure 2–3 Calculated Spectrum of Equivalent Source Pressure before and after Induced Failure.

revolution with a circular cross section. This model with a thin wall, as illustrated in Figure 2–6, will be utilized in the present analysis.

When the heart contracts, the apex is displaced to a new position due to the spiral nature of the muscle fibers. During ventricular motion the

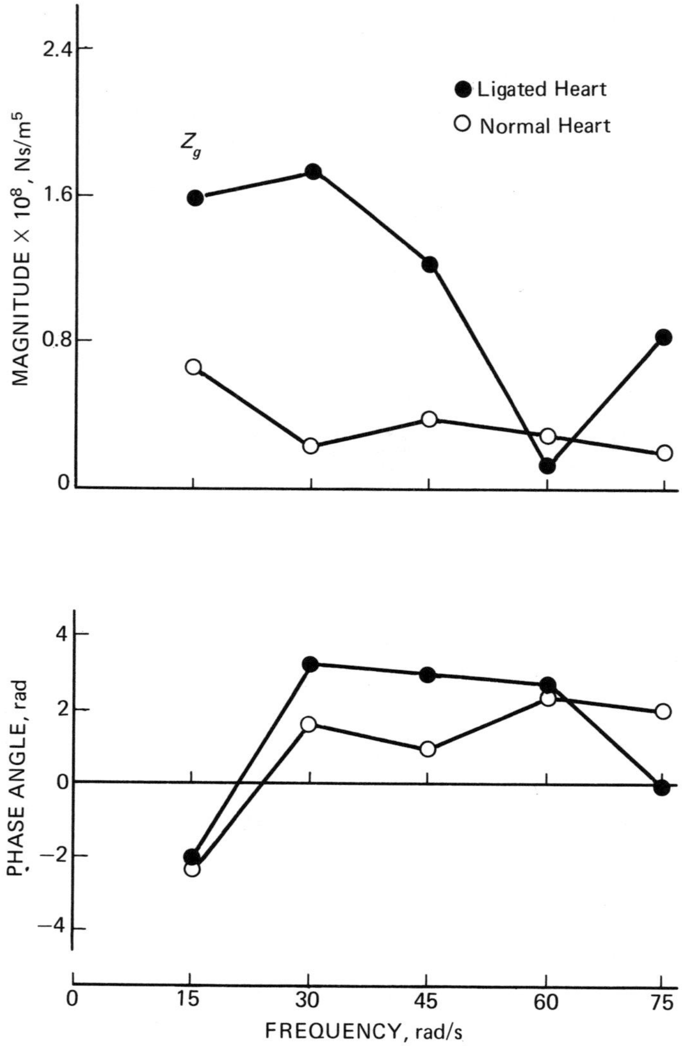

Figure 2–4 Calculated Source Impedance before and after Induced Failure.

septum separating the right and left ventricle is essentially in a fixed position. Therefore, the base-to-apex length of the left ventricle changes only slightly. Hawthorne (1961) has shown that in dogs this change is less than 4.5 percent. In the present analysis the base-to-apex length in the

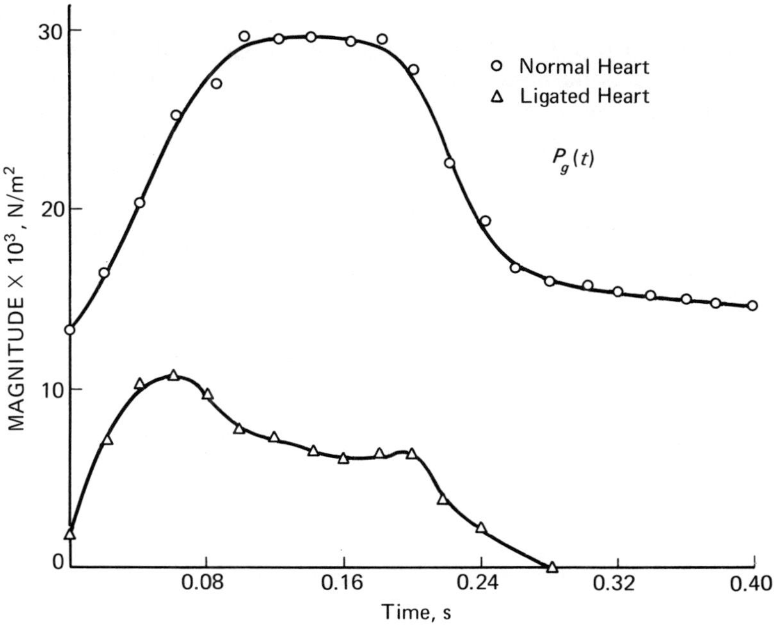

Figure 2–5 Time-Domain Representation of Equivalent Source Pressure before and after Induced Failure.

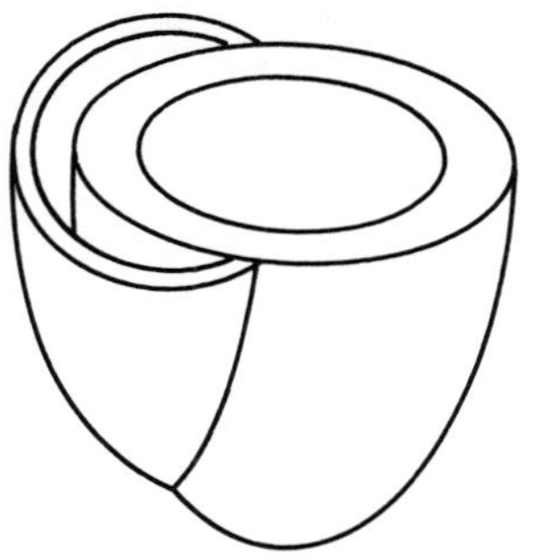

Figure 2–6 Ellipsoidal Model of the Left Ventricle.

semiellipsoidal model will be assumed constant. As shown by Sandler and Dodge (1963), very little error results from assuming that the wall thickness remains constant during the cardiac cycle. In the following shell model derivation this assumption will also be made.

Before we consider the ventricle geometry, it is important to choose an equation for muscle stress which later can be interrelated with ventricle geometry. For this purpose a form of Carlson's equation (1957) has been chosen and applied over the entire cardiac cycle. This approach was adopted by Robinson (1966), Shastri (1969), and Watts (1974). Min (1972) found little difference in his analysis of ventricular dynamics when he aternately used Carlson's equation only during isotonic contraction and Hill's equation (1938) during isovolumic contraction. In using this approach the active stress in a muscle segment is less than the isometric stress by an amount proportional to the rate of shortening of muscle:

$$\sigma(t) = \sigma_s - m\frac{dL(t)}{dt} \tag{2–7}$$

where $\sigma(t)$ = active stress as a function of time
σ_s = isometric stress (which can vary under physiological control and is a function of muscle length)
m = a constant
$L(t)$ = the muscle segment length as a function of time.

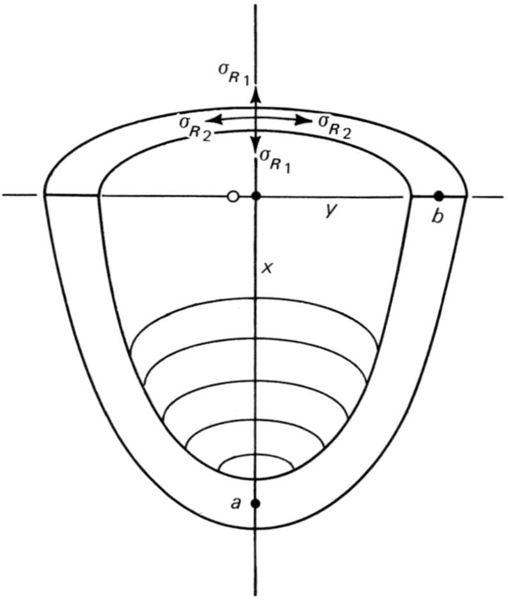

Figure 2–7 Section of the Shell Model of the Left Ventricle.

2.2.1 *Ellipsoidal Ventricle*

Consider the semiellipsoid shown in Figure 2–7. In this figure $\sigma_{R1}(t)$ and $\sigma_{R2}(t)$ are the longitudinal and circumferential stresses at $x = 0$, and x and y are coordinates corresponding to the major and minor axes. For this semiellipsoid the volume is given by

$$V_v = \frac{2}{3}\pi ab^2 \tag{2–8}$$

where $a =$ major semiaxis
$b =$ minor semiaxis

If muscle length of Eq. (2-7) is chosen as the greatest circumference of the ellipsoid, then

$$L(t) = 2\pi b(t) \tag{2–9}$$

If, in addition, the information about the constancy of the apical length is incorporated into the analysis, then the semiellipsoid volume as a function of time is given by

$$V_v(t) = BL^2(t) \tag{2–10}$$

where $B = a/(6\pi)$.

2.2.2 *Relationship between Wall Properties and Hydrodynamic Properties*

Laplace's equation for an ellipsoid which relates wall stress in a thin-walled shell to the internal pressure can be expressed as

$$\left(\frac{\sigma_{R1}}{R_1} + \frac{\sigma_{R2}}{R_2}\right) = \frac{P_v}{h_v} \tag{2–11}$$

where $R_1, R_2 =$ radii of curvature at the location of σ_{R1} and σ_{R2}
$P_v =$ left ventricular pressure
$h_v =$ left ventricular wall thickness (assumed uniform)

For an ellipsoid, $R_1 = a^2/b$ and $R_2 = b$. Measurements by Sandler and Dodge (1963) suggest that

$$R_1 \geqslant 4R_2 \tag{2–12}$$

and

$$\sigma_{R2} \geqslant 2\sigma_{R1} \tag{2–13}$$

Therefore, Eq. (2–11) can be expressed approximately as

$$\frac{\sigma_{R2}}{R_2} = \frac{P_v}{h_v} \tag{2–14}$$

or

$$\sigma_{R2} = \frac{bP_v}{h_v} \tag{2–15}$$

By averaging the circumferential stress over the entire semiellipsoid and defining this average stress as

$$\sigma_a = \frac{1}{a}\int_0^a \sigma(x)\,dx \tag{2–16}$$

it can be shown (Shastri 1969) that

$$\sigma_a = \frac{\pi}{4}\sigma_{R2} \tag{2–17}$$

As a function of time, therefore,

$$\sigma_a(t) = \frac{1}{8h_v}L(t)P_v(t) \tag{2–18}$$

Substituting Eq. (2–18) into Eq. (2–7) gives

$$P_v(t) = \frac{8h_v\sigma_s}{L(t)} - \frac{8h_v m}{L(t)}\left[\frac{dL(t)}{dt}\right] \tag{2–19}$$

If Eq. (2-10) is substituted into Eq. (2-19), then

$$P_v(t) = 8h_v\sqrt{B}\,\frac{\sigma_s}{\sqrt{V_v(t)}} - \frac{4h_v m}{V_v(t)}\left[\frac{dV_v(t)}{dt}\right] \tag{2–20}$$

2.3 Calculated Cardiac Parameters

2.3.1 *Stress-Volume Relationship*

Equation (2–4) can be expressed as a time-varying relationship of the following form:

$$P_v(t) = P_g(t) - Z_g(t) \cdot Q_a(t) \qquad (2\text{–}21)$$

A comparison of this equation with the shell model equation [Eq. (2–20)] yields the following relationship for ventricular volume:

$$V_v(t) = \frac{4h_v m}{Z_g(t)} \qquad (2\text{–}22)$$

Substituting this expression into Eq. (2–18), one finds that

$$\sigma_a(t) = \frac{1}{4}\left(\frac{m}{h_v B}\right)^{1/2} \frac{P_v(t)}{\sqrt{Z_g(t)}} \qquad (2\text{–}23)$$

The ventricular pressure $P_v(t)$ can be measured experimentally. In the discussion of an equivalent source representation of the left ventricle, it was shown that the phasor quantities P_g and Z_g can be obtained experimentally by loading the heart. Consequently, the time functions $P_g(t)$ and $Z_g(t)$ can also be obtained. By utilizing Eqs. (2–22) and (2–23) in conjunction with these experimentally deduced measurements, it is apparent that a curve relating stress (σ_a) and volume (V_v) can be obtained numerically. This curve should yield a reasonable representation of the Frank-Starling mechanism on a nondestructive basis. Therefore it could be a sensitive determiner of cardiac muscle status.

2.3.2 *End Diastolic Volume*

Equation (2–22) obviously can be utilized to determine the ventricular volume as a function of time and in particular to find its maximum value or end diastolic volume. It also can be used to estimate stroke volume and cardiac output. In order to carry out these numerical calculations, the constants h_v and m must be determined. The maximum value of the constant of the force-velocity relationship, m, can be determined from the work of Levine and Britman (1964) and is found to be $m = 1.5 \times 10^6$ Ns/m^3.

Shastri (1969) utilized this value and some measurements of ventricle wall thickness taken on an isolated heart to calculate end diastolic volume from pressure and flow measurements carried out on four dogs. His results are shown in Table 2–1. In his calculations stroke volume and cardiac output were obtained by integrating aortic flow rather than by using Eq. (2–22). Results useful for comparison were obtained by Taylor et al. (1967) on four dogs and are shown in Table 2–2.

2.3.3 *Isovolumic Stress*

By relating Eqs. (2–20) and (2–21) the calculated isovolumic stress σ_s can be shown to be

$$\sigma_s = \frac{1}{4}\left(\frac{m}{h_v B}\right)^{1/2} \frac{P_g(t)}{\sqrt{Z_g(t)}} \qquad (2\text{–}24)$$

Over a short period of time (one or two heart cycles) σ_s should be constant; however, over a longer period of time it is a controlled physiological function and will vary with physiological state.

2.3.4 *Maximum Muscle Velocity*

If one relates Eqs. (2–19) and (2–21), then it appears that muscle velocity in a circumferential direction is given by

$$V_m(t) = \frac{dL(t)}{dt} = \frac{1}{4}\left(\frac{m}{h_v B}\right)^{1/2} \sqrt{Z_g(t)} \cdot Q_a(t) \qquad (2\text{–}25)$$

Table 2–1
Volume Estimation

Dog Number	*Weight kg*	*Heart Rate, bpm*	*End Diastolic Volume, cm³*	*Stroke Volume, cm³*	*Stroke Volume ÷ End Diastolic Volume*	*Cardiac Output, l/min*
22	22	167	25	17.4	0.69	2.90
25	23	150	54	24.8	0.46	3.72
27	26	158	41	21.8	0.53	3.44
28	20	150	37	19.6	0.53	2.94

Source: Shastri (1969).

Table 2–2
Volume Estimation

Dog's Weight, kg	*Heart Rate, bpm*	*Stroke Volume ÷ End Diastolic Volume*	*Cardiac Output, l/min*
17.7	162	0.409	2.09
23	160	0.483	3.85
23.6	135	0.659	4.25
20.5	158	0.504	3.00

Source: Taylor et al. (1967).

By appropriately substituting the experimentally obtained values for $Q_a(t)$ and $Z_g(t)$, a relationship for muscle velocity as a function of time can be obtained. The maximum value of this function, then, is V_{max}, the maximum muscle velocity.

2.4 The Impaired Left Ventricle

Thus far indices have been developed for determining the status of the left ventricle based upon the assumption that the ventricle wall has uniform properties in both normal and abnormal situations. In many cases of impairment (for example, infarcts) the abnormality is localized, and the assumption of a uniform abnormality is unrealistic. The purpose of this section is to describe a mathematical model of the locally impaired left ventricle using a minimum number of restrictive assumptions. The description is of the development proposed by Watts (1974) in which the impaired ventricle is modeled as a multimesh circuit with varying elements depending upon the location and size of the impairment. Many of the assumptions needed in the mathematical development are the same as those used in the development of the uniform semi-ellipsoid shell model. These are:

1. Contraction is circumferential.
2. The left ventricle is a thin-walled shell.
3. The left ventricle is symmetric with inner and outer surfaces circular in cross section.
4. The wall thickness is constant in a plane orthogonal to the major axis.
5. Variations in wall thickness during systole are neglected.
6. Carlson's equation describes the muscle contraction.

There are some assumptions that are specific to this analysis. These are:

1. Muscle tissues contract independently and, within a limited area, synchronously.
2. Healthy tissue, when not contracting, can be described in terms of static elastic properties.
3. Impaired tissue can be considered elastic with an elastic modulus that increases with increasing stress.

The geometric approach to modeling taken in this section is to construct the left ventricle from a series of short cylindrical shells with radii determined by the overall geometry. Each shell is in general inhomogeneous, containing sections of both normal and impaired tissue. Equations governing the behavior of each shell are derived and the contributions of the several shells combined to determine the performance of the left ventricle.

The impaired heart is modeled in terms of three states. Two of these correspond to portions of the cardiac cycle. The third, the initial state, is used to define the ventricle in an unstressed condition, as a means for establishing initial values for geometric parameters. Only in this state is a geometric shape (an ellipsoid) assumed. This assumption is not necessary for the development, and the assumed shape could be replaced by measured dimensional data. The next state (state 1) describes the left ventricle after filling at the time of end diastolic pressure. In general, the shape is no longer ellipsoidal. State 1, which is a physiologically real state, has a static relationship to the initial state and can be used to derive reference dimensional data. The final state, state 2, describes conditions in the ventricle both during isovolumic contraction and after the aortic valve is open and blood is being pumped into the aorta. This last state could be split into two; but since it has been assumed that Carlson's equation describes muscle contraction during both isovolumic and isotonic contraction (see assumption 6), these are combined.

2.4.1 *Analysis of the Initial State*

If the initial state is chosen to be a semiellipsoid, as shown in Figure 2–8, then in cylindrical coordinates

$$\left(\frac{r}{b}\right)^2 + \left(\frac{z}{a}\right)^2 = 1 \tag{2–26}$$

and the volume enclosed by the shell is

$$V_v = \tfrac{2}{3}\pi ab^2 \tag{2–27}$$

By dividing this figure into N cylinders of equal length Δz, the incremental model of Figure 2–8 is obtained. This figure is composed of cylinders $C_1, C_2, \ldots, C_N$ with the radius of the jth cylinder given by

$$r_{vj} = b\sqrt{1 - \left(\frac{2j-1}{2N}\right)^2} \tag{2–28}$$

The volume of this approximation to the ellipsoid, V_a, is given by

$$V_a = \pi b^2 \sum_{j=1}^{N} \left[1 - \left(\frac{2j-1}{2N}\right)^2\right]\frac{a}{N} \tag{2–29}$$

This is equal to

$$V_a = \frac{2}{3}\pi b^2 a\left(1 + \frac{1}{8N^2}\right) \tag{2–30}$$

Each cylinder consists of a contractile section of length l_1 and an impaired section of length l_2, as shown in Figure 2–9. Since each cylinder may contain an arbitrarily designated impaired section, the total impaired area can assume any desired shape.

2.4.2 *Analysis of the Left Ventricle at End Diastole*

In this state, the cylindrical segments are described in terms of their passive elastic properties. The elasticities of normal and impaired tissues are assumed to differ. The shape of the left ventricle is determined by the extent and shape of the impaired section as well as by its elasticity relative to the unimpaired tissue.

The following list of symbols is used for the subsequent derivations:

$l_1 =$ length of unimpaired segment of ventricle (initial state)
$l_2 =$ length of impaired segment of ventricle (initial state)
$l_{11} =$ length of unimpaired segment of ventricle at end diastole
$l_{12} =$ length of impaired segment of ventricle at end diastole
$l_1(t) =$ length of unimpaired segment of ventricle during systole
$l_2(t) =$ length of impaired segment of ventricle during systole
$r_{vj} =$ radius of jth segment of ventricle
$r_{v1j} =$ radius of jth segment of ventricle at end diastole
$r_{vj}(t) =$ radius of jth segment of ventricle during systole
$\Delta l_1 =$ change in length of unimpaired segment of ventricle between states 1 and 0 $(l_{11} - l_1)$
$\Delta l_2 =$ change in length of impaired segment of ventricle between states 1 and 0 $(l_{12} - l_2)$
$\Delta l_2(t) =$ change in length of impaired segment of ventricle, relative to l_2, during systole
$h_v =$ ventricle wall thickness in initial state
$h_{v1} =$ ventricle wall thickness of unimpaired segment in state 1
$h_{v2} =$ ventricle wall thickness of impaired segment in state 1
$E_{v1} =$ elasticity of unimpaired ventricle wall at end diastole
$E_{v2} =$ elasticity of impaired ventricle wall at end diastole
$E'_{v2} =$ elasticity of impaired ventricle wall during systole
$P_0 =$ end diastolic pressure
$p_v(t) =$ left ventricular pressure
$\sigma_1 =$ stress in unimpaired heart muscle segment
$\sigma_2 =$ stress in impaired heart muscle segment

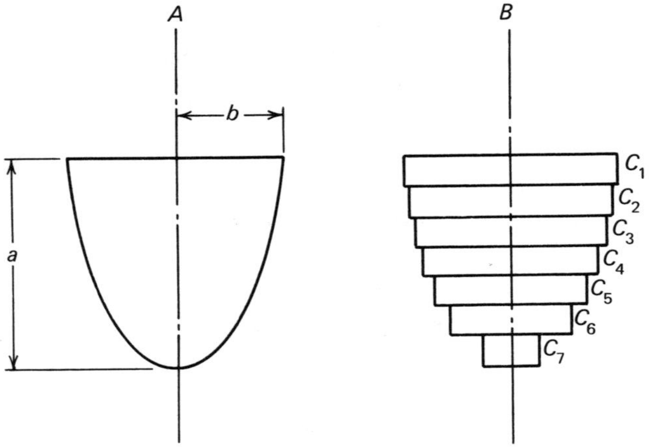

Figure 2–8 Ventricular Models.

From Figure 2–9, the relationship between force, tension, and stress in a cylindrical segment can be seen to be

$$F_\theta = \sigma_1 A = \sigma_1 h_{v1} \Delta z \tag{2–31}$$

and

$$T_\theta = \frac{F_\theta}{\Delta z} = \sigma_1 h_{v1} \tag{2–32}$$

Since the tension throughout the uniform-width cylinder must be constant,

$$T_\theta = \sigma_1 h_{v1} = \sigma_2 h_{v2} \tag{2–33}$$

If the thickness of muscle in a section is approximately equal to h_v, then Eq. (2–33) can be expressed as

$$T_\theta = h_v E_{v1} \frac{\Delta l_1}{l_1} = h_v E_{v2} \frac{\Delta l_2}{l_2} \tag{2–34}$$

Laplace's equation for a cylinder implies that

$$\frac{T_{\theta j}}{r_{v1j}} = P_0 \tag{2–35}$$

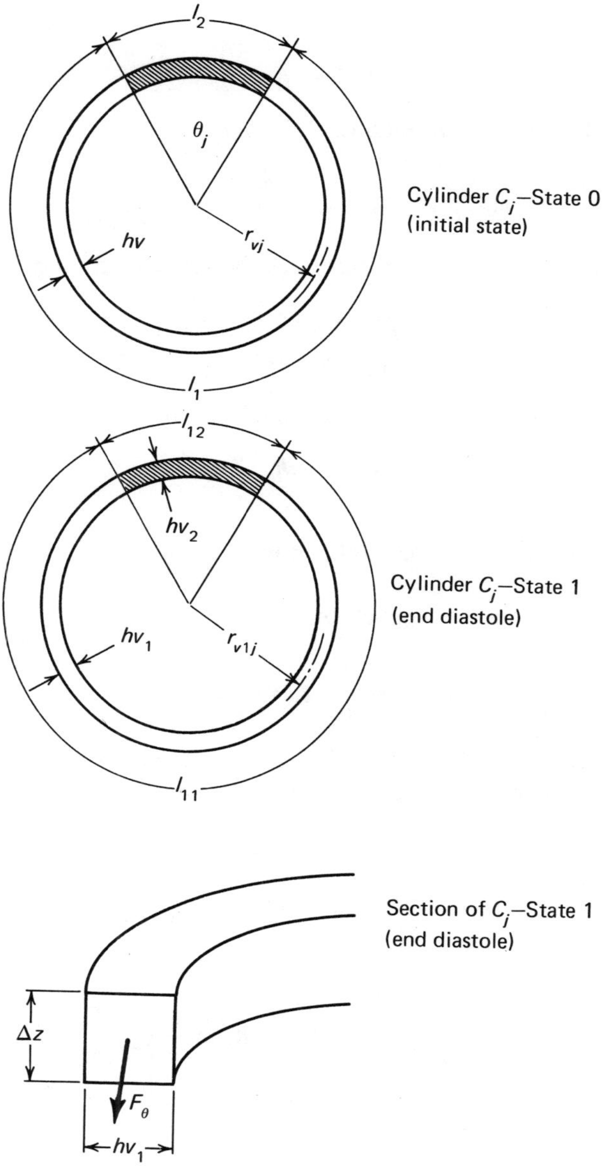

Figure 2–9 Cylindrical Section of Incremental Ventricular Model.

By definition

$$2\pi r_{v1j} = l_1 + l_2 + \Delta l_1 + \Delta l_2 \tag{2–36}$$

and

$$2\pi r_{vj} = l_1 + l_2 \tag{2–37}$$

Combining Eqs. (2–34) through (2–37) gives

$$r_{v1j} = \frac{r_{vj}}{1 - P_0/(2\pi h_v)(l_1/E_{v1} + l_2/E_{v2})} \tag{2–38}$$

Substituting Eq. (2–28), which describes the segmented model, yields

$$r_{v1j} = \frac{(b/2N)[4N^2 - (2j-1)^2]^{1/2}}{1 - P_0/(2\pi h_v)(l_1/E_{v1} + l_2/E_{v2})} \tag{2–39}$$

Equations (2–38) and (2–39) have a singularity if

$$\frac{l_2}{E_{v2}} = \frac{2\pi h_v}{P_0} - \frac{l_1}{E_{v1}} \tag{2–40}$$

The model would have to be modified in the event that this condition were approximated.

End diastolic volume is given by

$$V_0 = \sum_{j=1}^{N} \pi r_{v1j}^2 \Delta z \tag{2–41}$$

The values of r_{v1j} can be obtained from Eq. (2–39). An alternate solution can be obtained by reference to Figure 2–9, where

$$l_2 = r_{vj}\theta_j \tag{2–42}$$

$$l_1 = (2\pi - \theta_j)r_{vj} \tag{2–43}$$

Letting

$$K = \frac{P_0}{h_v E_{v1}} \quad \text{and} \quad K_1 = \frac{E_{v1} - E_{v2}}{2\pi E_{v2}} \tag{2–44}$$

then

$$V_0 = \pi b^2 a \sum_{j=1}^{N} \frac{\frac{1}{N}\left|1 - \left(\frac{2j-1}{2N}\right)^2\right|}{\left[1 - Kb(1 + K_1\theta_j)\sqrt{1 - \left(\frac{2j-1}{2N}\right)^2}\right]^2} \tag{2–45}$$

As N becomes large, $\theta_j \rightarrow \theta(z)$ and $r_j \rightarrow r_v(z)$. If $\theta(z)$ and $r_v(z)$ are continuous functions, then end diastolic volume is given by

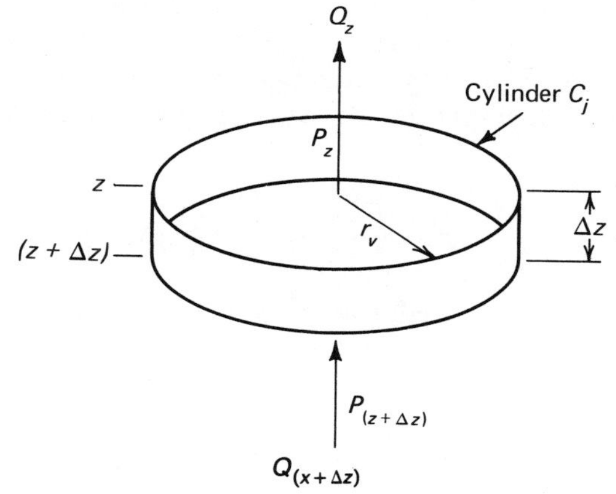

Figure 2–10 Pressures and Flows at Incremental Cylindrical Section.

$$V_0 = \pi \int_0^a \left[\frac{r_v(z)}{1 - K[1 + K_1 \theta(z)] r_v(z)} \right]^2 dz \qquad (2\text{–}46)$$

2.4.3 Analysis of the Left Ventricle during Contraction

This state, state 2, includes both isovolumic contraction, during which no blood is being pumped into the aorta, and approximately isotonic contraction, when the aortic valve is open and blood is pumped into the aorta. The energy for pumping is supplied by the healthy contractile tissue. The model remains in state 2 until the pressure in the aorta exceeds the left ventricular pressure, at which time the aortic valve closes and the left ventricle relaxes to be filled from the left atrium. The relaxed left ventricle is assumed to fill passively at constant pressure (end diastolic pressure) in returning to state 1. The equations governing contraction must include acceleration of the blood, stretching of the impaired tissue, viscous forces, and contractile muscle mechanics.

Consider an incremental cylindrical section as shown in Figure 2–10. Applying continuity concepts and Newton's law gives

$$\Delta Q = -\frac{\partial A}{\partial t} \Delta z \qquad (2\text{–}47)$$

and

$$\Delta F = \left[k(A) Q + \rho \frac{\partial Q}{\partial t} \right] \Delta z \qquad (2\text{–}48)$$

where ΔF and ΔQ are the force across the cylinder and the incremented flow produced by radial contraction of the cylindrical shell. The coefficient $k(A)$, a function of geometry, determines the viscous component of force because of flow. If flow through the cylinder obeys Poiseuille's law, then Eq. (2–48) becomes

$$\Delta F = \left[\frac{8\pi\nu}{A}Q + \rho\frac{\partial Q}{\partial t}\right]\Delta z \tag{2–49}$$

In the notation being used, Carlson's equation, modified to express the tension developed by a strip of active tissue, is given by

$$T = T_s + m_1\frac{dl_1(t)}{dt} \tag{2–50}$$

The tension throughout the section is constant; therefore

$$T = \frac{E'_{v2}h_v}{l_2}\Delta l_2(t) \tag{2–51}$$

If the following substitutions are made:

$$C_v = \frac{E'_{v2}h_v}{l_2} \tag{2–52}$$

$$L = l_1(t) + l_2(t) \tag{2–53}$$

then

$$T = T_s + m_1\frac{d}{dt}[L - \Delta l_2(t)] \tag{2–54}$$

and

$$T = C_v\Delta l_2(t) \tag{2–55}$$

Equations (2–54) and (2–55) can be combined using a series expansion to yield

$$T = \sum_{n=0}^{\infty}\left(-\frac{m_1}{C_v}\frac{\partial}{\partial t}\right)^n T_s - C_v\sum_{p=1}^{\infty}\left(-\frac{m_1}{C_v}\frac{\partial}{\partial t}\right)^p L \tag{2–56}$$

Since $L = 2\pi r_v$,

$$T = \sum_{n=0}^{\infty}\left(-\frac{m_1}{C_v}\frac{\partial}{\partial t}\right)^n T_s - 2\pi C_v\sum_{p=1}^{\infty}\left(-\frac{m_1}{C_v}\frac{\partial}{\partial t}\right)^p r_v \tag{2–57}$$

The first term of Eq. (2–49) is nonlinear but is small in magnitude. For this equation it can be assumed that A remains constant during systole. If we let $8\pi v/a = K_v$, then

$$\Delta F = \left(K_v Q + \rho \frac{\partial Q}{\partial t}\right)\Delta z \tag{2–58}$$

which is a linear equation between ΔF andQ. By definition

$$F = PA = \pi r_v^2 P \tag{2–59}$$

Combining Eqs. (2–57), (2–59), and (2–35) (Laplace's equation) yields

$$F = \pi r_v \sum_{n=0}^{\infty} \left(-\frac{m_1}{C_v}\frac{\partial}{\partial t}\right)^n T_s - 2\pi^2 r_v C_v \sum_{p=1}^{\infty} \left(-\frac{m_1}{C_v}\frac{\partial}{\partial t}\right)^p r_v \tag{2–60}$$

Equation (2–47) can be rewritten as

$$\Delta Q = -2\pi r_v \Delta z \frac{\partial r_v}{\partial t} \tag{2–61}$$

The nth time derivative of ΔQ in terms of r_v, then, is

$$\frac{d^n(\Delta Q)}{dt^n} = -\pi \Delta z \sum_{j=0}^{n+1} \binom{n+1}{j} \frac{\partial^j r_v}{\partial t^j} \cdot \frac{\partial^{n+1-j} r_v}{\partial t^{n+1-j}} \tag{2–62}$$

If one defines the series

$$S(\Delta Q) = K \sum_{n=0}^{\infty} k^n \frac{\partial^n(\Delta Q)}{\partial t^n} \tag{2–63}$$

where K and k are arbitrary constants, then

$$S(\Delta Q) = -\pi K \Delta z \sum_{n=0}^{\infty} k^n \sum_{j=0}^{n+1} \binom{n+1}{j} \frac{\partial^j r_v}{\partial t^j} \cdot \frac{\partial^{n+1-j} r_v}{\partial t^{n+1-j}} \tag{2–64}$$

Neglecting the products of derivatives

$$S(\Delta Q) \cong -\pi K \Delta z \sum_{n=0}^{\infty} \left[k^n \binom{n+1}{0} r_v \frac{\partial^{n+1} r_v}{\partial t^{n+1}} + \binom{n+1}{n+1} \frac{\partial^{n+1} r_v}{\partial t^{n+1}} r_v\right] \tag{2–65}$$

or

$$S(\Delta Q) \cong -2\pi K \Delta z r_v \sum_{n=0}^{\infty} k^n \frac{\partial^{n+1} r_v}{\partial t^{n+1}} \tag{2–66}$$

Equation (2–66) may be rewritten as

$$\frac{S(\Delta Q)}{\Delta z} \cong -2\pi \frac{K}{k} r_v \sum_{p=1}^{\infty} \left(k \frac{\partial}{\partial t}\right)^p r_v \tag{2–67}$$

Comparing Eq. (2–67) with Eq. (2–60) and letting $k = -m_1/C_v$ and $K = \pi m_1$, we get

$$F = \pi r_v \sum_{n=0}^{\infty} \left(-\frac{m_1}{C_v}\frac{\partial}{\partial t}\right)^n T_s + \frac{S(\Delta Q)}{\Delta z} \tag{2–68}$$

or alternately

$$F = \pi\left[r_v \sum_{n=0}^{\infty} \left(-\frac{m_1}{C_v}\frac{\partial}{\partial t}\right)^n T_s - m_1 \sum_{n=0}^{\infty} \left(-\frac{m_1}{C_v}\frac{\partial}{\partial t}\right)^n \frac{\Delta Q}{\Delta z}\right] \tag{2–69}$$

Equations (2–47) through (2–69) deal with the jth cylinder. In order to model different cylindrical sections and the array of cylindrical sections that make up the entire ventricle, subscripts for each separate cylinder will be utilized in the remaining equations.

Let

$$G_j(t) = \pi r_{vj}(t) T_s \tag{2–70}$$

Taking the Laplace transform of Eq. (2–69) and substituting Eq. (2–52) and Eq. (2–70), we get

$$F_j(s) = \frac{G_j(s)}{1 + (m_1 l_2/E'_{v2} h_v)s} - \frac{\pi m_1 [\Delta Q_j(s)/\Delta z]}{1 + (m_1 l_2/E'_{v2} h_v)s} \tag{2–71}$$

Taking the Laplace transform of Eq. (2–58) yields

$$\Delta F_j(s) = [K_{vj} Q_j(s) + \rho s Q_j(s)]\Delta z \tag{2–72}$$

The circuit analog to Eqs. (2-70) to (2-72) for the jth cylinder is shown in Figure 2–11. By relating the circuit diagram to the equations, it can be seen that the circuit elements have the values

$$L_{sj} = \rho \tag{2–73}$$

$$R_{sj} = K_{vj} = \frac{8\pi\nu}{A_j} \tag{2–74}$$

$$R_{pj} = \pi m_1 \tag{2–75}$$

$$c_{pj} = \frac{l_{2j}}{\pi E'_{v2j} h_v} \tag{2–76}$$

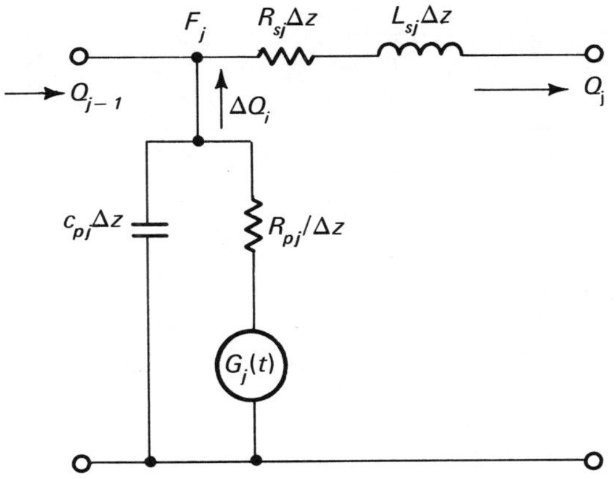

Figure 2–11 Network Analog Model for Incremental Cylindrical Section.

The parallel capacitive element for each cylinder is determined entirely by the impaired tissue, in particular its length and elasticity. The series-resistive element and the generator output are both dependent upon the radius of the cylindrical section.

The circuit equivalent for a complete left ventricle during contraction can be obtained by combining the equivalent circuits for N strips. This network is shown in Figure 2–12. In this figure the aortic valve is represented by a diode, and the aortic input impedance is represented by an equivalent network with initial force conditions. The overall equivalent circuit represents the impaired left ventricle during its contractile state. Since the electrical analog is a ladder network, it can be readily analyzed by using existing computer circuit analysis programs.

2.4.4 Applications of Impaired Left Ventricle Model

By collecting data widely from the literature on canine hearts, Watts (1974) was able to evaluate the parameters needed to carry out the calculations suggested by the model. He segmented the ventricle into ten cylinders and evaluated parameters (both geometric and elastic) for each of these. The elasticity of the impaired tissue (infarct region) was not easily determined and, in fact, was found to vary with different experimental subjects. Therefore he selected three values for the calculations: 3.16 times unimpaired tissue, equal to unimpaired tissue, and a factor of 3.16 below unimpaired tissue. The accompanying curves show some calculated results for healed post-ereolateral infarcts. Figure 2–13 shows the effect of impairment size on end

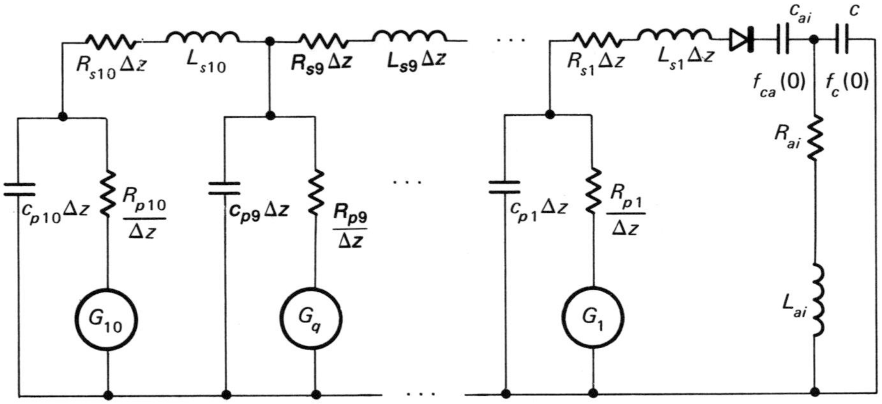

Figure 2–12 Network Analog Model of Left Ventricle during Systole Pumping into the Aorta through the Aortic Valve.

diastolic volume with a fixed end diastolic pressure of 4 mm Hg. The impairment chosen was approximately circular in shape. Curves for the three values of impaired tissue elasticity (high, medium, low) are shown. In Figure 2–14 the effect of impairment on stroke volume is presented for the same end diastolic pressure and impaired tissue elasticities. As is well known, end diastolic pressure often increases in cases of myocardial infarction in order to increase the stroke volume. The calculated effect of this increase on end diastolic volume is shown in Figure 2–15 for a 20 percent area infarct. For the same infarct, the effect of increasing end diastolic pressure on the calculated stroke volume is shown in Figure 2–16. Finally, for the low-elasticity impaired tissue, the ventricular bulging that is often observed in certain impairments is shown in the calculations illustrated in Figure 2–17.

It is apparent from these results that calculations using the derived model of the impaired left ventricle demonstrate many of the physiological phenomena observed with myocardial infarcts.

References

Carlson, F.D., "Kinematic Studies of Mechanical Properties of Muscles," in J.W. Remington (ed.), *Tissue Elasticity*, American Physiological Society, Washington, D.C., 1957.

Eggleton, R.C.; Townsend, C.; Herrick, J.; Templeton, G.; and Mitchell, J.H., "Ultrasonic Visualization of Left Ventricular Dynamics," *IEEE Trans. on Sonics and Ultrasonics* 17 (1970): 143–53.

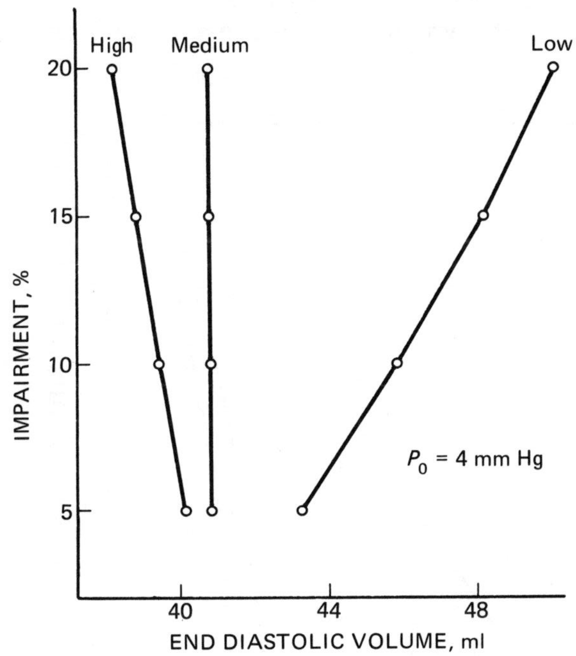

Figure 2–13 Variation of End Diastolic Volume with Impairment Size.

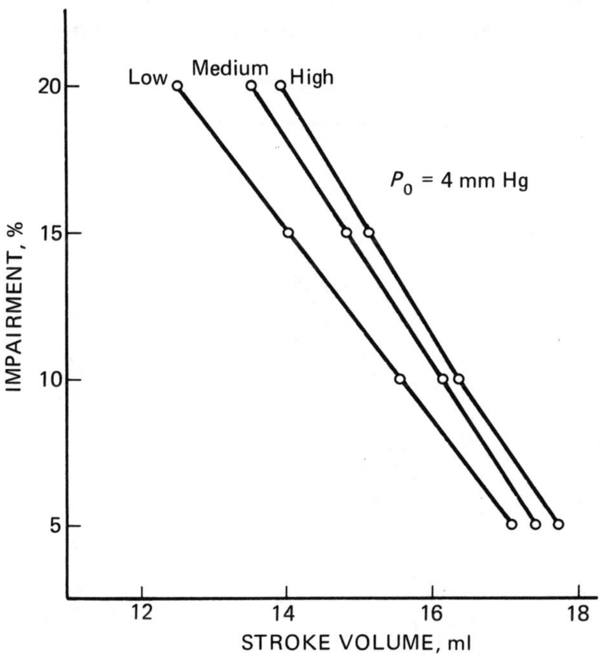

Figure 2–14 Effect of Impairment Size on Stroke Volume.

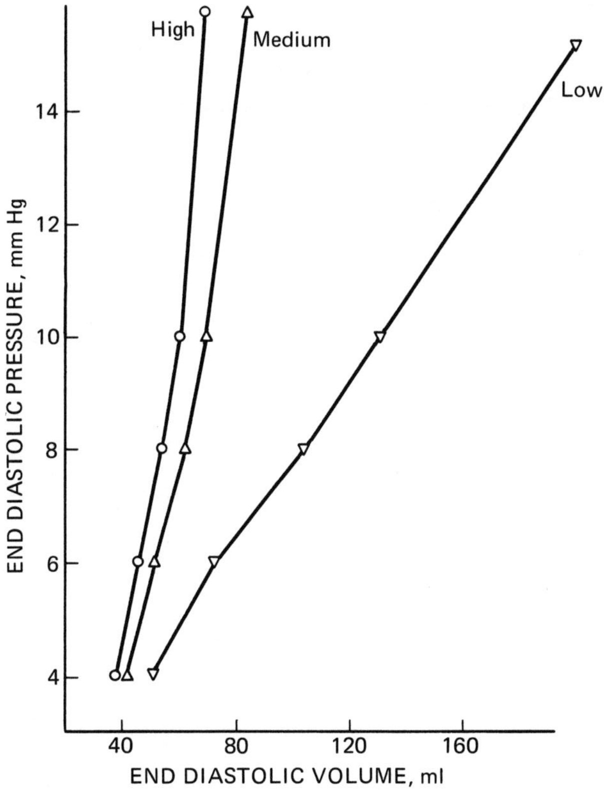

Figure 2–15 Relationship between End Diastolic Pressure and End Diastolic Volume (20 percent Infarction).

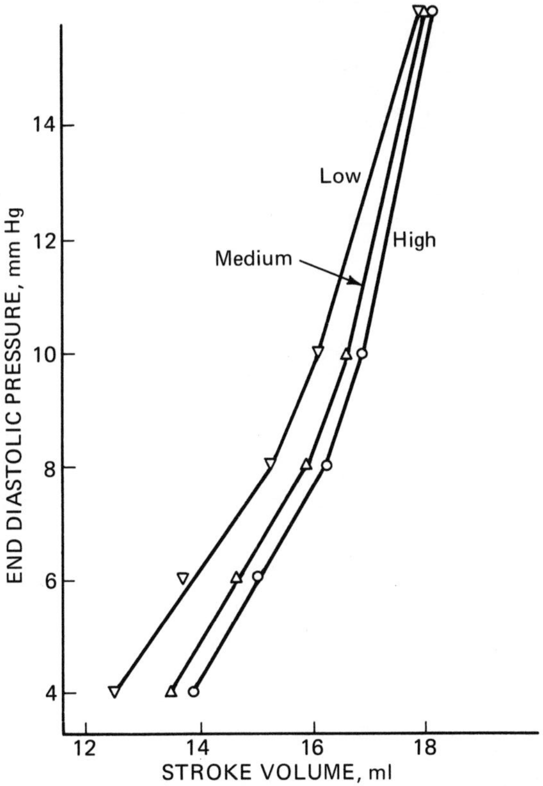

Figure 2–16 Relationship between Stroke Volume and End Diastolic Pressure (20 percent Infarction).

Fich, S.; Welkowitz, W.; Shastri, S.; Jaron, D.; and Kantrowitz, A., "An Equivalent Pressure Source for the Heart," *Int. J. Eng. Sci.* 11 (1973): 601–11.

Hawthorne, E.W., "Instantaneous Dimensional Changes of the Left Ventricle in Dogs," *Circ. Res.* 9 (1961): 110.

Hill, A.V., "Heat of Shortening and Dynamic Constants of Muscle," *Proc. Roy. Soc.* (*Biol.*) *series B* 126 (1938): 136–95.

Hood, W.P., et al., "Comparison of Calculation of Left Ventricular Wall Stress in Man from Thin-Walled and Thick-Walled Ellipsoidal Models," *Circ. Res.* 24 (1969): 576.

Katz, A.M., and Brady, H.J., "Mechanical and Biochemical Correlates of Cardiac Contraction (1)," *Modern Concepts of Cardiovascular Disease*, 40 (1971): 39–43.

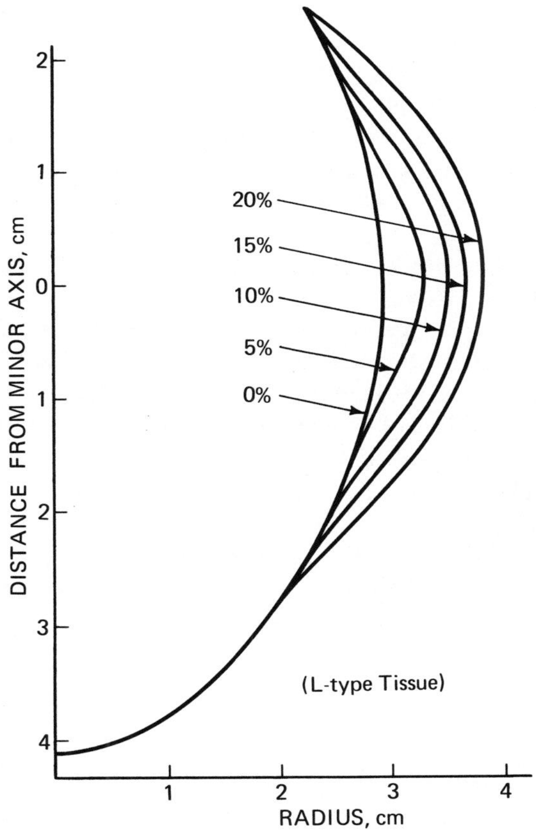

Figure 2–17 Shape of Left Ventricle at End Diastolic Pressure as a Function of Impairment (EDP = 8 mm Hg).

Koushanpour, E., and Collings, W.D., "Validation and Dynamic Applications of an Ellipsoid Model of the Left Ventricle," *J. Appl. Physiol.* 21 (1966): 1655.

Levine, H.J., and Britman, N.A., "Force-Velocity Relations in the Intact Dog Heart," *J. Clin. Invest.* 43 (1964): 1383.

Min, B.G., "Analysis and Optimization of Cardiac Assistance by Intra-aortic Balloon Pumping," Ph.D. thesis, Rutgers University, New Brunswick, N.J., 1972.

Noordergraaf, A., and Meester, G.T., "Hemodynamics and the Heart," *Bibl. Cardiol.* 30 (1973): 75–86.

Puri, N.N., and Gido, J.T., "Control Systems for Circulatory Assist Devices," University City Science Center, Philadelphia, 1968, pp. 3–11.

Robinson, D.A., "Quantitative Analysis of the Control of Cardiac Output in the Isolated Left Ventricle," *Circ. Res.* 17 (1966): 207.

Rushmer, R.F., *Cardiovascular Dynamics*, 2d ed., W.B. Saunders Co., Philadelphia, 1961.

Sandler, H., and Dodge, H.T., "Left Ventricular Tension and Stress in Man," *Circ. Res.* 13 (1963): 91.

Shastri, S.J., "A Thevenin Equivalent Model of the Left Ventricle Derived from Hemodynamic Measurements Obtained by Use of a Ventricular Assist Pump," Ph.D. thesis, Rutgers University, New Brunswick, N.J., 1969.

Talbot, S.A., and Gessner, U., *Systems Physiology*, John Wiley & Sons, New York, 1973, pp. 376–96.

Taylor, R.R., et al., "A Quantitative Analysis of Left Ventricular Myocardial Function in the Intact, Sedated Dog" *Circ. Res.* 21 (1967): 99.

Van Den Bos, G.C.; Elzinga, G.; Westerhof, N.; and Noble, M.I., "Problems in the Use of Indices of Myocardial Contractility," *Cardiovasc. Res.* 7 (1973): 834–48.

Vayo, H.W., "The Motion of the Left Ventricle," *Bull. Math. Biophys.* 28 (1966): 355.

Watts, R.N., "A Mathematical Model for Studying the Mechanical Properties of the Impaired Left Ventricle," Ph.D. thesis, Rutgers University, New Brunswick, N.J., 1974.

3 Properties of a Tapered Aorta

Second to the heart itself, the aorta, which is the major conduit of blood from the heart to the systemic circulation, may well be the most important organ in the circulatory system. One of the distinctive characteristics of blood flow in the aorta is the change in shape of the pressure and flow pulses during propagation from the heart to the periphery of the vascular system. Because these shape changes must be implicitly related to the physical characteristics of the system, there has been an extensive research effort expended to explain these changes and to obtain a clear understanding of the mechanics of the blood flow process. These changes in shape have been variously attributed to wave reflections from the peripheral system, damping, and arterial wall resonances (Rushmer 1961). Since the pressure pulse increases in amplitude and the flow pulse decreases in amplitude during propagation along the aorta, there has been emphasis on the reflection theory to explain the changes in waveshape (McDonald 1960; Talbot 1973). This reasoning is based upon the consideration of an analogous electrical transmission line with standing waves. Such a line has regions with increasing voltage amplitudes and decreasing current amplitudes. One of the earliest alternatives to the reflection theory was offered by Taylor (1964) who proposed a nonuniform propagation velocity mechanism to characterize the wave propagation. Models using nonuniform wave propagation theory are based upon many known physical characteristics of the aorta such as its tapering area (Fry, Griggs, and Greenfield 1964), nonuniform elasticity (Patel, Greenfield, and Fry 1964), and visco-elastic wall structure (Bergel 1964).

Following Taylor's work, the investigation of the nonuniform wave propagation characteristics of the aorta has been greatly extended (Fich, Welkowitz, and Hilton 1966; Hilton, Fich, and Welkowitz 1966; Welkowitz and Fich 1967; Strano 1969; Strano, Welkowitz, and Fich 1972; Welkowitz, Fich, and Strano 1972). In this chapter the hemodynamic relationships between the presure and flow of blood in the aorta are studied by considering fluid mechanical equations for a thin-walled tapered tube of nonuniform properties. The emphasis in this solution is on the effects of the geometric tapering and of the elastic nonuniformities. Some consideration is given also to elastic nonlinearities. In order to concentrate on the effects of the nonuniformities, the mathematical models chosen are usually nonreflective. The question of reflection from the periphery, however, is considered in some detail. Approximate solutions are obtained for the complex sets of equations arising from these investigations by using methods developed for nonuniform transmission line analysis. By employing a parameter identification and optimization technique in conjunction with the mathematical models of the aorta, and with pressure measurements obtained in the aorta by means of catheterization, it has been possible to calculate physical properties of the aorta such as diameter, taper, and wall elasticity. This technique presently is being studied for its applicability to the diagnosis of arterial diseases.

It should be emphasized that many assumptions have been made in the various mathematical models presented in this chapter. The major ones are that the blood vessel wall can be represented as a thin elastic tube, that variations of parameters in the radial direction are negligible in their effects on the propagated waves and therefore the system is representable by one-dimensional differential equations, and that the aorta is approximately terminated by a nonreflective mechanical impedance.

3.1 Theoretical Analysis

In order to derive reasonable, distributed-parameter mathematical models of blood vessel sections, it is necesary to consider the basic physical laws that govern hydrodynamic flow, i.e., conservation of matter and conservation of momentum. Starting with such general considerations and then making reasonable assumptions, one can arrive at desired mathematical models with a clear understanding of the simplifications used.

Initially, the blood can be thought of as a compressible fluid which obeys the relationship (Streeter 1961)

$$d\rho = \frac{\rho}{\beta} dP \tag{3–1}$$

where $\rho =$ blood density at a point along the aorta
$P =$ blood pressure at that point
$\beta =$ bulk modulus of elasticity of blood

As indicated, the blood vessel is being considered as a thin-walled tube so that a differential section can assumed to follow Laplace's law. This can be expressed approximately as

$$dA_a = \frac{A_a}{E(h_a/2R_i)} dP \tag{3–2}$$

where $A_a =$ cross-sectional area at a point along the aorta
$h_a =$ vessel wall thickness at that point
$R_i =$ inside radius of the vessel at that point
$E =$ modulus of elasticity of the vessel wall at that point

From the equation of continuity (conservation of matter), using conventional coordinates, we get

$$-\frac{\partial(\rho Q)}{\partial x}dx = \frac{\partial(\rho A_a)}{\partial t}dx \tag{3–3}$$

where Q is the total blood flow at a point along the aorta.

If we apply the principle of conservation of momentum to the differential section, then approximately

$$-\frac{\partial(\rho A_a)}{\partial x}dx - \frac{8\pi\nu}{A_a}Q\,dx = \frac{\partial(\rho Q)}{\partial t}dx + \frac{\partial(\rho Q^2/A_a)}{\partial x}dx \tag{3–4}$$

where ν is the viscosity of the blood.

The basic thesis of this chapter is that the properties of the aorta are heavily dependent upon its geometric and elastic nonuniformities (or taper). Therefore the differential section considered in deriving Eqs. (3–2), (3–3), and (3–4) must be tapered. The equations presented involve some approximations when applied to a tapered section. The numerical values applicable to the problem being considered—blood flow in a tapered aorta—make these approximations reasonable. Streeter, Keitzer, and Bohr (1964) in considering the problem of a geometrically tapering aorta also justified some of these assumptions. It should be pointed out that further approximations will be required for the simplifications used to put these equations in a form suitable for solution.

Equation (3–3) can be expanded and combined with Eqs. (3–1) and (3–2) to yield

$$-\frac{\partial Q}{\partial x} - \frac{Q}{\beta}\frac{\partial P}{\partial x} = \left[\frac{A_a}{E(h_a/2R_i)} + \frac{A_a}{\beta}\right]\frac{\partial P}{\partial t} \tag{3–5}$$

Since blood is relatively incompressible (β is very large), Eq. (3–5) becomes approximately

$$-\frac{\partial Q}{\partial x} = \frac{A_a}{E(h_a/2R_i)}\frac{\partial P}{\partial t} \tag{3–6}$$

Equation (3–4) can be expanded and combined with Eqs. (3–1) and (3–2), and when terms in $1/\beta$ are eliminated, the resultant equation is

$$-\frac{\partial P}{\partial x}\left[1 + \frac{P}{E(h_a/2R_i)}\right] = \frac{\rho}{A_a}\frac{\partial Q}{\partial t} + \frac{Q}{A_a^2}\left(8\pi\nu + 2\rho\frac{\partial Q}{\partial x} - \frac{\rho Q}{A_a}\frac{\partial A_a}{\partial x}\right) \tag{3–7}$$

In considering the numerical values applicable to the aorta, the second term on the left-hand side of the equation is negligible compared to the first and can be dropped. The last two terms on the right-hand side of the equation, while sometimes smaller than the Poiseuille term, are not negligible. The approach taken in this development has been to lump the latter three terms into an "effective viscosity" term so that the final momentum equation becomes

$$-\frac{\partial P}{\partial x} = \frac{\rho}{A_a}\frac{\partial Q}{\partial t} + \frac{8\pi\nu_{\text{eff}}}{A_a^2}Q \tag{3–8}$$

where ν_{eff} combines the effects of the energy loss terms.

The coefficients of the variables of Eqs. (3–6) and (3–8) depend upon the distance along the aorta and may also vary with pressure. For ease in applying electrical analogies to arrive at solutions to these equations, it is convenient to express them in the form of the telegrapher's equations:

$$-\frac{\partial Q}{\partial x} = C_a\frac{\partial P}{\partial t} \tag{3–9}$$

and

$$-\frac{\partial P}{\partial x} = L_a\frac{\partial Q}{\partial t} + R_a Q \tag{3–10}$$

where

$$\begin{aligned} C_a &= A_a/E(h_a/2R_i) \\ L_a &= (\rho/A_a) \\ R_a &= 8\pi\nu_{\text{eff}}/A_a^2 \end{aligned}$$

An examination of L_a, C_a, and R_a indicates that they vary with different powers of the spatially dependent parameters. Therefore, the standard methods of solution for nonuniform transmission lines do not apply. A number of special approximation methods have been studied for solving Eqs. (3–9) and (3–10) in terms of their applicability to the blood flow problem.

3.1.1 *Conical Taper with Nonlinear Elasticity*

It has been pointed out that the bulk modulus of elasticity of blood is very large; therefore the variation in blood density is very small. Thus, it is reasonable to consider that $\rho = \rho_0$, a constant. The inertance of the blood then becomes

$$L_a = \frac{\rho_0}{A_a} \tag{3–11}$$

From Eq. (3–2) the area as a function of pressure can be expressed as

$$A_a = A_{a0}\left[1 + \frac{P - P_0}{E(h_a/2R_i)}\right] \tag{3–12}$$

where A_{a0} = area at the time of end diastolic pressure
P_0 = end diastolic pressure

Lawton (1955) has indicated that the dynamic modulus of elasticity of the blood vessel wall varies with stretch. From Eq. (3–12) this implies that the modulus of elasticity also varies with pressure. Since the amount of stretch is relatively small, one possible assumption is that the variation of the elastic constant with pressure is approximately linear with a form

$$E = E_0[1 + k_E(P - P_0)] \tag{3–13}$$

The diameter of the aorta tapers appreciably. In the present analysis it is assumed that this taper is conical and that the area at diastole as a function of distance along the aorta can be expressed as

$$A_{a0} = A_{a0}(0)(1 - k_A x) \tag{3–14}$$

The elastin content of the blood vessel wall varies with location along the aorta, and in particular it increases as one moves distally along the aorta (Patel, Greenfield, and Fry 1964). It is assumed that this variaton is linear and that the elastic constant has the form

$$E_0 = E_0(0)(1 + k_T x) \tag{3–15}$$

If it is further assumed that the aorta is terminated nonreflectively (Fich et al. 1970), then Eqs. (3–9) through (3–15) can be utilized to solve for the propagated waveshapes of pressure and flow in the aorta using difference equations and numerical integration. The difference equations have the from

$$-\frac{\Delta Q_x}{\Delta x} = C_a \frac{\Delta P_t}{\Delta t} \tag{3–16}$$

$$-\frac{\Delta P_x}{\Delta x} = L_a \frac{\Delta Q_t}{\Delta t} + R_a Q \tag{3–17}$$

The subscript x represents an increment with distance and the subscript t represents an increment with time. Since it has been assumed that there is no reflected wave, initial curves of pressure and flow at the aortic root in numerical form can be utilized with Eqs. (3–16) and (3–17) to obtain new time function curves at a distance Δx. This process can then be repeated for each successive interval Δx. Equations (3–12) and (3–13) can be employed to obtain the time variations of E and A_a, and furthermore these time functions can be obtained for any location along the aorta.

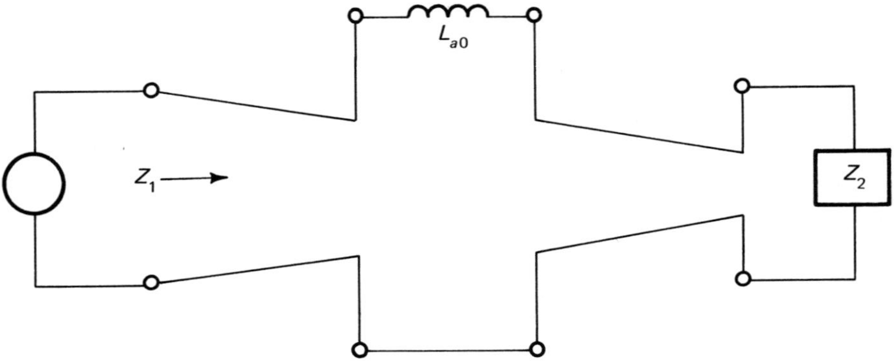

Figure 3–1 Schematized Aorta with Lumped Inertance.

3.1.2 A Nonuniform Hybrid Model

The numerical procedure presented in the previous section, while capable of generating pressure and flow waveforms along the aorta and incorporating other than conical aorta geometries, cannot provide the understanding of the propagation problem (and the possibility of determining aorta parameters from simple measurements) that a closed form mathematical solution can. As has been pointed out, however, standard solution techniques for Eqs. (3–9) and (3–10) are not applicable because of the differences in dependence of L_a, C_a, and R_a on aorta diameter.

An approximation approach that has been successful in making the problem tractable to analytical solution is described in this section. First, following a procedure that has been used experimentally on telephone lines, the distributed inertance can be replaced by a lumped inertance located at the center of the schematized aorta, as shown in Figure 3–1. The distributed portions of the schematized system now have equations

$$-\frac{\partial Q}{\partial x} = C_a \frac{\partial P}{\partial t} \tag{3–18}$$

$$-\frac{\partial P}{\partial x} = R_a Q \tag{3–19}$$

Second, the taper of the aorta can be approximated by an exponential geometry (Attinger, Anne, and Sugawara 1965). If the origin is taken at the distal end, the geometry of a massless tapered section is diagramed in Figure 3–2. The inside radius of this schematized aorta is

$$r_a(x) = r_{a2}\, e^{kx/2} \tag{3–20}$$

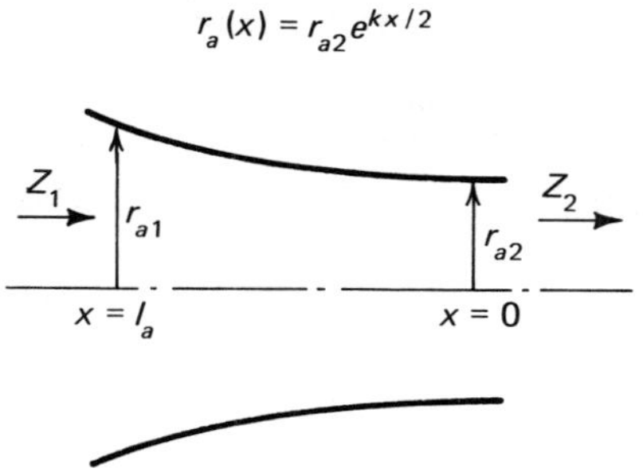

Figure 3–2 Exponentially Tapered Aorta.

Third, the hydraulic capacitance of Eq. (3–18) can be defined as

$$C_a = \frac{dA_a}{dP} = \frac{2A_a(x)r_a(x)}{E(x)h_a} \tag{3–21}$$

Since the modulus of elasticity of the vessel wall has been shown to increase as one moves distally from the heart (Apter 1965), it will be assumed that

$$E(x) = \frac{E_{a2}}{r_a(x)} \tag{3–22}$$

or

$$E(x) = \frac{E_{a2}}{r_{a2}}e^{-kx/2} \tag{3–23}$$

in the coordinate system of Figure 3–2. Since $A_a(x) = \pi r_a(x)^2$, the hydraulic capacitance is

$$C_a = \left(\frac{2\pi}{E_{a2}h_a}\right)r_a(x)^4 \tag{3–24}$$

Equation (3–21) can be expressed as

$$C_a = \frac{dA_a}{dr_a}\cdot\frac{dr_a}{dP} = 2\pi r_a\frac{dr_a}{dP} \tag{3–25}$$

By using experimentally determined data (Patel et al. 1963) for dr_a/dP and using Eq. (3–20) for r_a, the hydraulic capacitance C_a of Eq. (3–25) agrees very well with the relationship of Eq. (3–24), as shown in Figure 3–3. This figure tends to support both the relationship for hydraulic capacitance given in Eq. (3–24) and the assumed relationship for the modulus of elasticity given in Eq. (3–22).

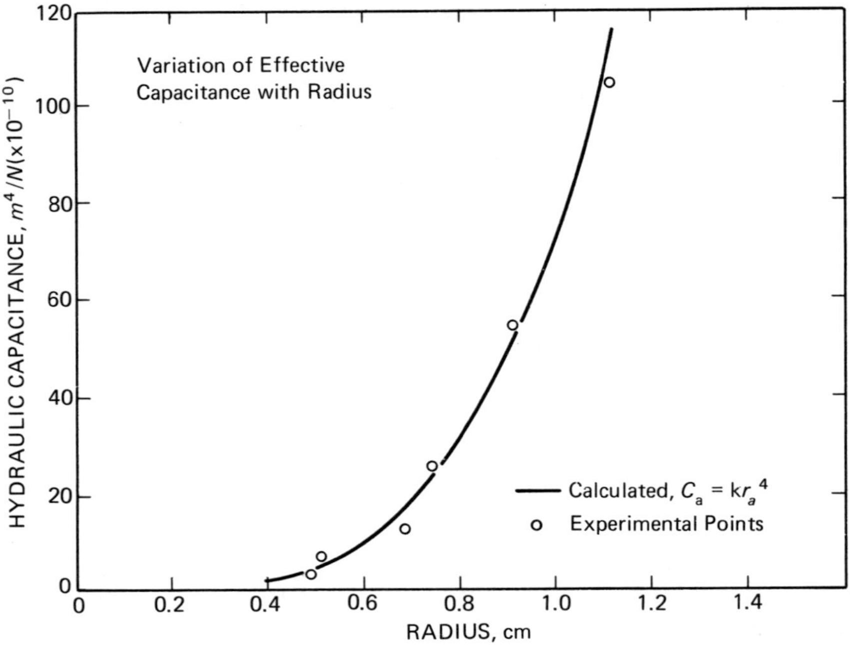

Figure 3–3 Variation of Effective Capacitance with Radius.

By using Eq. (3–20), the hydraulic resistance can be expressed as

$$R_a = \left(\frac{8\nu_{\text{eff}}}{\pi r_{2a}{}^4}\right)e^{-2kx} \tag{3–26}$$

From Eq. (3–24) the hydraulic capacitance is

$$C_a = \left(\frac{2\pi r_{a2}{}^4}{E_{a2}h_a}\right)e^{2kx} \tag{3–27}$$

Therefore,

$$R_a C_a = \frac{16\nu_{\text{eff}}}{E_{a2}h_a} \tag{3–28}$$

which is a constant independent of x.

Under these conditions, it is now possible to solve Eqs. (3–18) and (3–19) and to combine the solution with the lumped inertance characteristic in order to obtain pressure and flow transfer functions for any sectional length of aorta.

Assuming initial quiescence, the Laplace transforms of Eqs. (3–18) and (3–19) are

$$\frac{d}{dx}Q(x,s) = sC_a(x)P(x,s) \tag{3–29}$$

$$\frac{d}{dx}P(x,s) = R_a(x)Q(x,s) \tag{3–30}$$

Combining these equations, the transformed differential equation for the pressure is

$$\frac{d^2}{dx^2}P(x,s) = sR_a(x)C_a(x)P(x,s) + \frac{1}{R_a(x)}\frac{d}{dx}P(x,s)\left[\frac{d}{dx}R_a(x)\right] \tag{3–31}$$

If one defines $R_{a2} = 8\nu_{\text{eff}}/(\pi r_{a2}{}^4)$ and $C_{a2} = 2\pi r_{a2}{}^4/(E_{a2}h_a)$, then

$$\frac{d^2}{dx^2}P(x,s) + 2k\frac{d}{dx}P(x,s) - sR_{a2}C_{a2}P(x,s) = 0 \tag{3–32}$$

The solution of this equation is

$$P(x,s) = e^{-kx}(K_1 \cosh \gamma x + K_2 \sinh \gamma x) \tag{3–33}$$

where $\gamma = (k^2 + sR_{a2}C_{a2})^{1/2}$ and $K_1 = P(0,s) = P_2$. In a similar manner, one can obtain a solution for the flow, $Q(x,s)$. If the terminating impedance is defined as

$$Z_2 = \frac{P(0,s)}{Q(0,s)} \tag{3–34}$$

then K_2 is expressable in terms of Z_2. If we define

$$P_2 = P(0,s) \tag{3–35}$$

$$Q_2 = Q(0,s) \tag{3–36}$$

$$P_1 = P(l_a,s) \tag{3–37}$$

$$Q_1 = Q(l_a,s) \tag{3–38}$$

then

$$P_1 = e^{-kl_a}\left(\cosh \gamma l_a + \frac{k}{\gamma}\sinh \gamma l_a\right)P_2 + \left(\frac{R_{a2}}{\gamma}e^{-kl_a}\sinh \gamma l_a\right)Q_2 \tag{3–39}$$

$$Q_1 = \left[\frac{(\gamma^2 - k^2)}{\gamma R_{a2}}e^{kl_a}\sinh \gamma l_a\right]P_2 + \frac{e^{kl_a}}{\gamma}(\gamma \cosh \gamma l_a - k \sinh \gamma l_a)Q_2 \tag{3–40}$$

In the transformed notation this solution is of the form

$$P_1(s) = A_T(s)P_2(s) + B_T(s)Q_2(s) \tag{3–41}$$

$$Q_1(s) = C_T(s)P_2(s) + D_T(s)Q_2(s) \tag{3–42}$$

where the transmission coefficients A_T, B_T, C_T, and D_T are obtainable from Eqs. (3–39) and (3–40). For this massless section of the aorta, the pressure and flow transfer functions are given by

$$T_P = \frac{P_2}{P_1} = \frac{1}{A_T + (B_T/Z_2)} = \frac{e^{kl_a}}{\cosh \gamma l_a + (1/\gamma)(k + R_{a2}/Z_2)\sinh \gamma l_a} \tag{3–43}$$

$$T_q = \frac{Q_2}{Q_1} = \frac{1}{C_T Z_2 + D_T} = \frac{e^{-kl_a}}{\cosh \gamma l_a + (1/\gamma)[(\gamma^2 - k^2)(Z_2/R_{a2}) - k]\sinh \gamma l_a} \tag{3–44}$$

The input impedance to the massless section is given by

$$Z_1 = \frac{P_1}{Q_1} = \frac{e^{-2kl_a}\left[\cosh \gamma l_a + \frac{1}{\gamma}\left(k + \frac{R_{a2}}{Z_s}\right)\sinh \gamma l_a\right]}{\frac{1}{Z_2}\cosh \gamma l_a + \left(\frac{\gamma}{R_{a2}} - \frac{k^2}{\gamma R_{a2}} - \frac{k}{\gamma Z_2}\right)\sinh \gamma l_a} \tag{3–45}$$

In terms of the schematized aorta of Figure 3–1, if the aorta is considered reflectionless at its periphery, then the distal section must be reflectionless. Under this condition

$$Z_2 = \frac{R_{a2}}{\gamma - k} \tag{3–46}$$

Refer to Figure 3–1: the inertance of the blood can be taken into account in the solution for pressure and flow wave transmission by calculating an overall transmission matrix using standard matrix multiplication techniques.

$$\begin{vmatrix} A_T & B_T \\ C_T & D_T \end{vmatrix} = \begin{vmatrix} A_{T1} & B_{T1} \\ C_{T1} & D_{T1} \end{vmatrix} \times \begin{vmatrix} 1 & sL_0 \\ 0 & 1 \end{vmatrix} \times \begin{vmatrix} A_{T2} & B_{T2} \\ C_{T2} & D_{T2} \end{vmatrix} \tag{3–47}$$

The inertance parameter, L_0, is given by

$$L_{a0} = \frac{\rho l_a}{A_{\text{av}}} \tag{3–48}$$

where l_a is the length of aorta section being considered and A_{av} is the average area for this section. The matrix $[A_{T1}\, B_{T1}\, C_{T1}\, D_{T1}]$ represents the transmission characteristics of the proximal half of the aorta (assumed massless), and the values can be obtained from Eqs. (3–39) and (3–40) with $l_a/2$ substituted for l_a. The matrix $[A_{T2}\, B_{T2}\, C_{T2}\, D_{T2}]$ represents the transmission characteristics of the distal half of the aorta, and again values can be obtained from Eqs. (3–39) and (3–40) with $l_a/2$ substituted for l_a. The value of R_{a2} is different for the two matrices.

The validity of this model of the aorta has been investigated by taking a measured input pressure wave and calculating a derived output pressure wave, a derived input impedance, a derived input flow wave, and a derived output flow wave. These derived quantities can then be compared to measured values. This procedure and its results are discussed in detail in Section 3.2. If the input pressure is a steady-state pulsatile wave, then the complex frequency parameter s in the equations becomes purely imaginary and is equal to $j\omega$. The input waveform can then be broken down into its harmonics and calculations carried out for each harmonic. The derived waves can be subsequently synthesized from the calculated harmonics.

3.1.3 A Network Equivalent for the Nonuniform Hybrid Aorta Model Input Impedance

In some applications of circulatory system models, such as the study of left ventricle dynamics presented in Chapter 2, it is convenient to represent the aorta and peripheral systemic circulation as an equivalent network characterized by its input impedance. Using Eqs. (3–39), (3–40), (3–45), and (3–46) and considering the input ventricular pressure to be pulsatile steady state, Watts (1974) has shown that the input impedance to the aorta as a function of frequency is given by

$$Z_1(j\omega) = \frac{\gamma R_{a1}\, e^{(\gamma+k)l_a} + \dfrac{j\omega L_{a0}}{2}(\gamma - k)^2 - \dfrac{L_{a0} R_{a1} C_{a1}}{2}\omega^2 e^{\gamma l_a}}{(\gamma - k)\left[\gamma e^{(\gamma+k)l_a} - \dfrac{L_{a0} C_{a1}}{2}\omega_2\left(e^{\gamma l_a} - 1\right)\right]} \tag{3–49}$$

Equation (3–49) represents the input impedance of the hybrid aorta model that has been presented. A third-order lumped circuit equivalent to Z_1 can be synthesized from the general form

$$\hat{Z}_1(j\omega) = K_1 \frac{-\omega^2 + jK_2\omega + \omega_1^2}{j\omega(-\omega^2 + jK_3\omega + \omega_2^2)} \tag{3–50}$$

For the network shown in Figure 3–4 this becomes

$$\hat{Z}_1(j\omega) = \frac{C_{ai} + C}{jC_{ai}C\omega}\left[\frac{-\omega^2 + j\dfrac{R_{ai}}{L_{ai}}\omega + \dfrac{1}{L_{ai}(C_{ai} + C)}}{-\omega^2 + j\dfrac{R_{ai}}{L_{ai}}\omega + \dfrac{1}{L_{ai}C}}\right] \qquad (3\text{–}51)$$

Values for ω_1 and ω_2 can be obtained from inspection of the plot of $|Z_1(j\omega)|$ versus ω for physiologically appropriate constants. In addition, at high frequencies

$$\lim_{\omega\to\infty} Z_1, \hat{Z}_1 = 0 \qquad (3\text{–}52)$$

while at low frequencies

$$\lim_{\omega\to 0} Z_1(\omega) = \lim_{\omega\to 0} \hat{Z}_1(\omega) \qquad (3\text{–}53)$$

From these conditions, Watts (1974) determined that

$$C_{ai} = 0.467 \times 10^{-9} \text{ m}^5/\text{N}$$
$$C = 1.27 \times 10^{-9} \text{ m}^5/\text{N}$$
$$L_{ai} = 1.32 \times 10^5 \text{ Ns}^2/\text{m}^5$$
$$R_{ai} = 3.57 \times 10^6 \text{ Ns/m}^5$$

By using these values, the amplitude and phase of the input impedance of the lumped network of Figure 3–4 as compared to the same functions for the hybrid nonuniform model with appropriate physiological parameters are shown in Figures 3–5 and 3–6. It can be seen from these figures that the simple circuit of Figure 3–4 is a good representation of the hybrid

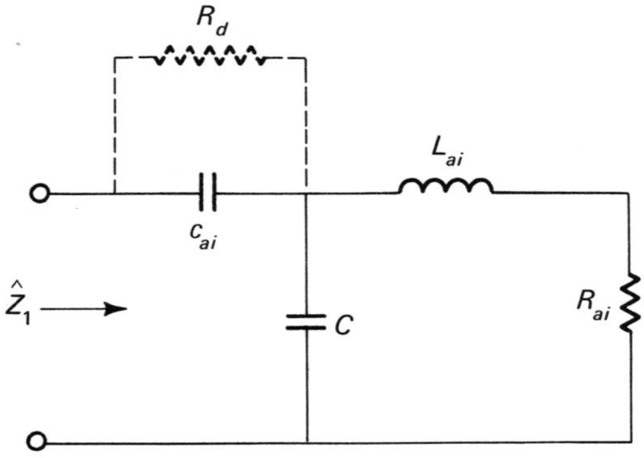

Figure 3–4 Network Equivalent for Hybrid Aorta Model.

distributed model of the aorta over the physiologically useful range of frequencies.

3.2 Verification of Theoretical Description

In Section 3.1 a number of methods of modeling the characteristics of a nonuniform aorta were presented. All these methods involve many approximations in their derivations; therefore it is necessary to compare model predictions concerning pressure and flow wave propagation with information obtained from the literature of blood circulation or measured experimentally.

In order to carry out model calculations for any of the models, it is necessary to have values for the diferential equation coefficients, for example, the values of R_a, L_a, and C_a of Eqs. (3–9) and (3–10). This in turn requires the knowledge of various physical parameters of the blood and the aorta. An examination of the definitions of R_a, L_a, and C_a suggests that one

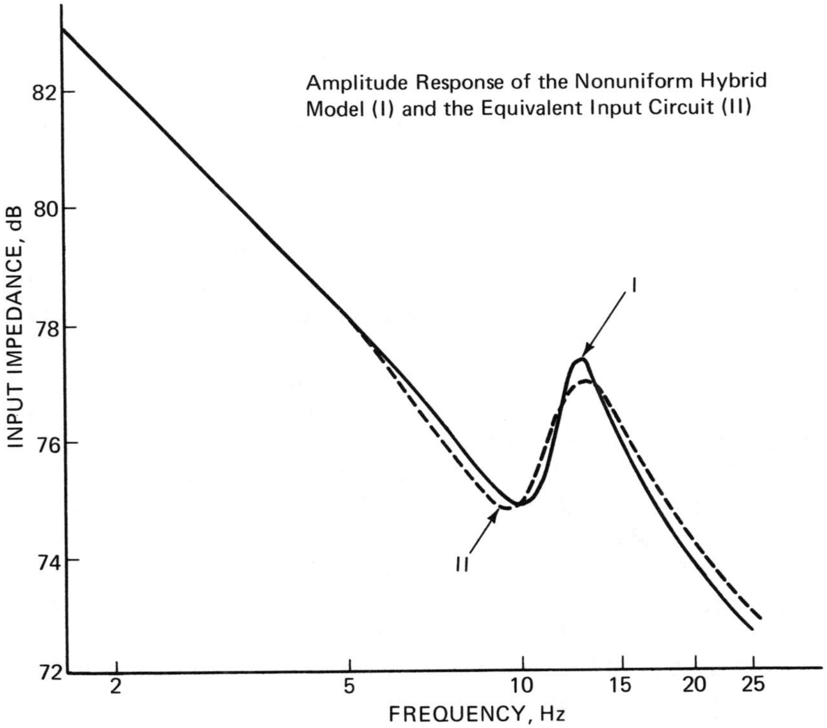

Figure 3–5 Amplitude Response of Input Impedance for Nonuniform Hybrid Model and Equivalent Network.

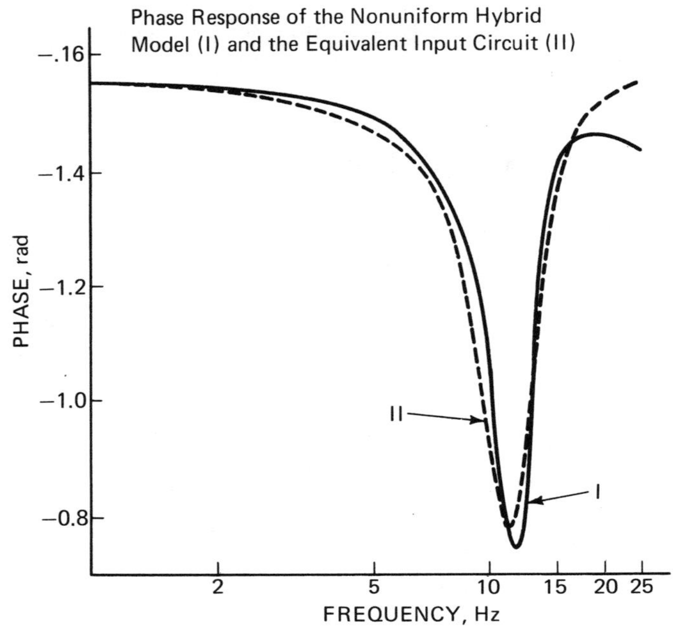

Figure 3–6 Phase Response of Input Impedance for Nonuniform Hybrid Model and Equivalent Network.

needs to know blood density, blood viscosity, and a loss factor to compute effective blood viscosity, diameter, wall thickness, and elastic modulus of the aorta, as well as the variations of these quantities along the aorta. The values of the physical parameters of blood are as follows (McDonald 1960): blood density is approximately equal to 1005 kg/m^3, and blood viscosity is approximately 0.004 Ns/m^2. Measurements of hydraulic resistance by Fry, Griggs, and Greenfield (1964) suggest that losses in pulsatile blood flow are 10 to 40 times as great as the expected simple viscous losses due to Poiseuille flow. It is therefore reasonable to assume a value for ν_{eff} of between 0.04 and 0.16 Ns/m^2. In the models considered, these values were assumed uniform throughout the aortic section.

The geometric parameters of the aorta naturally vary widely with the size of the subject. However, ascending aorta cross-sectional areas of 3×10^{-4} to $6 \times 10^{-4}\,\text{m}^2$ are reasonable for adult humans, and between 2×10^{-4} and $4 \times 10^{-4}\,\text{m}^2$ for adult dogs between 15 and 30 kg in weight (Rushmer 1961; Patel et al. 1963). Measurements of elastic modulus and thickness-to-diameter ratio vary depending upon species, specific experimental subject, and location along the aorta (McDonald 1960; Bergel 1964;

Patel et al. 1963). Rushmer (1961) presents a reasonable value in the ascending aorta of $h_a/2R_i = 0.08$. Elastic moduli for the same location appear to vary from about 0.5×10^5 to $5.0 \times 10^5 \mathrm{N/m^2}$.

Since $(Eh_a/2R_i)$ appears as a composite constant in the definition of hydraulic capacitance, a value for this composite parameter (which will be called β_e) is a most useful quantity. Patel, Greenfield, and Fry (1964) define a quantity E_p as

$$E_p = \frac{\Delta P}{\Delta r_a} \cdot r_a \tag{3–54}$$

By comparing Eq. (3–54) with Eq. (3–25), it can be seen that

$$\beta_e = \tfrac{1}{2} E_p \tag{3–55}$$

If we use the values of Patel, Greenfield, and Fry (1964) for E_p in the ascending aorta of human and dog, then

$$\beta_e(\text{human}) = 3.9 \times 10^4 \mathrm{N/m^2}$$

and

$$\beta_e(\text{dog}) = 4.0 \times 10^4 \mathrm{N/m^2}$$

Specific numerical values pertinent to each model were chosen within the framework of values discussed above and are presented in the discussion of verification of each model.

3.2.1 Model with Conical Taper and Nonlinear Elasticity

Verification of this model was carried out using values from McDonald (1960) for typical pressure and flow curves as a function of distance along the aorta. These curves are shown in Figure 3–7. The parameter values selected were considered reasonable for human pulsatile blood flow and are shown in Table 3–1. The input excitation pressure wave used was a typical curve from Rushmer (1961) measured in the ascending aorta. With this input excitation and Eqs. (3–11) through (3–17), Figure 3–8 shows calculated pressure waveforms at locations along the aorta, Figure 3–9 shows calculated flow waveforms along the aorta, and Figure 3–10 shows cross-sectional area variations.

In comparing the calculated curves of Figures 3–8 and 3–9 with Figure 3–7, it can be seen that the shape changes of the pressure and flow waveforms tend to follow the propagation characteristics that have been generally measured. These include an increase in the pressure peak, a

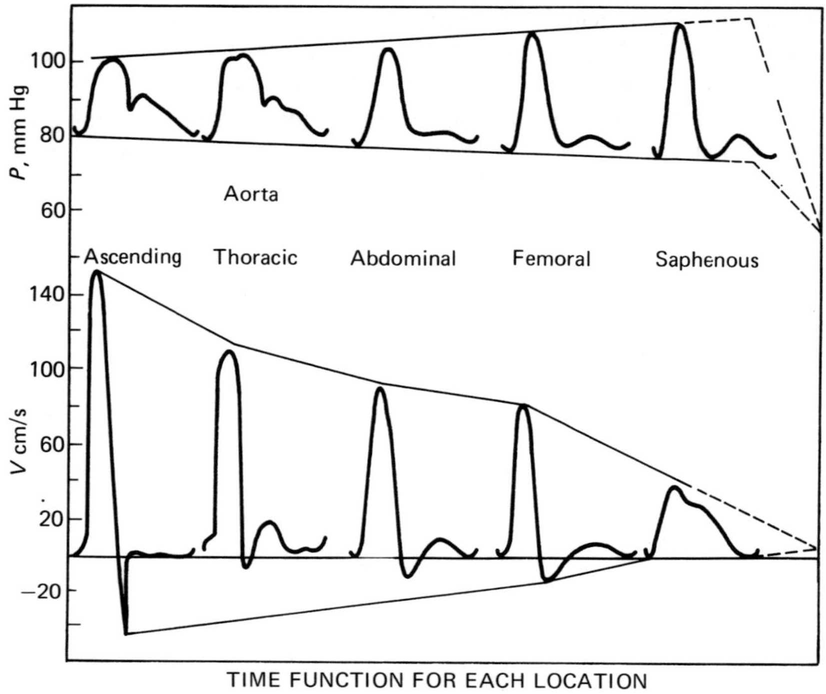

Figure 3–7 Pressure and Flow Waveforms along the Aorta.

Table 3–1
Physical Parameters for Verification of Model with Conical Taper and Nonlinear Elasticity

Parameter, Unit	*Value*
Blood density, kg/m^3	1005
Effective blood viscosity, Ns/m^2	0.04
Heart rate, bpm	75
Ascending aorta, cross-sectional area, m^2	4×10^{-4}
$h_a/2Ri$	0.08
Elastic modulus in ascending aorta, N/m^2	2.0×10^5
Variation of elastic modulus in ascending aorta from diastolic to systolic pressure	11%
Length of aorta section for calculations, m	0.3
Aorta cross-sectional area at end of section length, m^2	2.8×10^{-4}
Elastic modulus at end of section length, N/m^2	4.0×10^5

sharpening up of this peak, and the development of the dichrotic wave. Along with the changes in the pressure waveform, the amplitude of the flow pulse decreases markedly, and the backflow component becomes smaller.

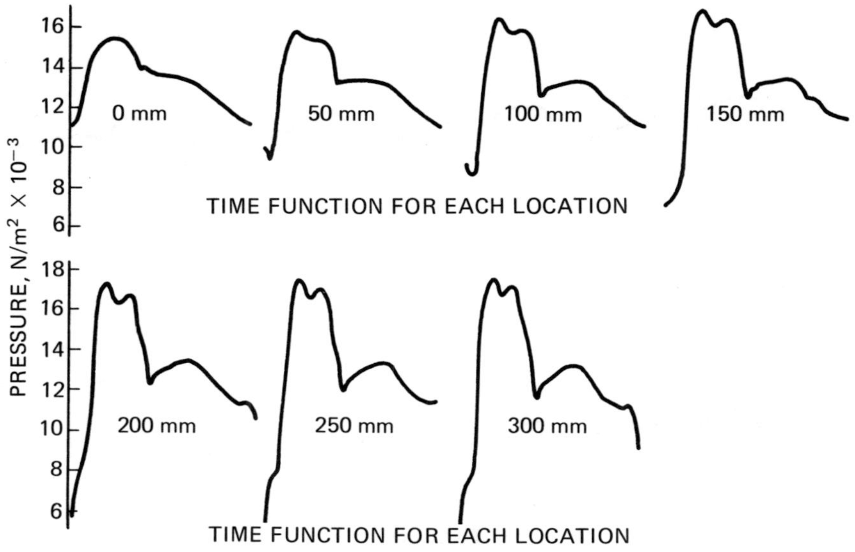

Figure 3–8 Calculated Pressure Waveforms along the Aorta.

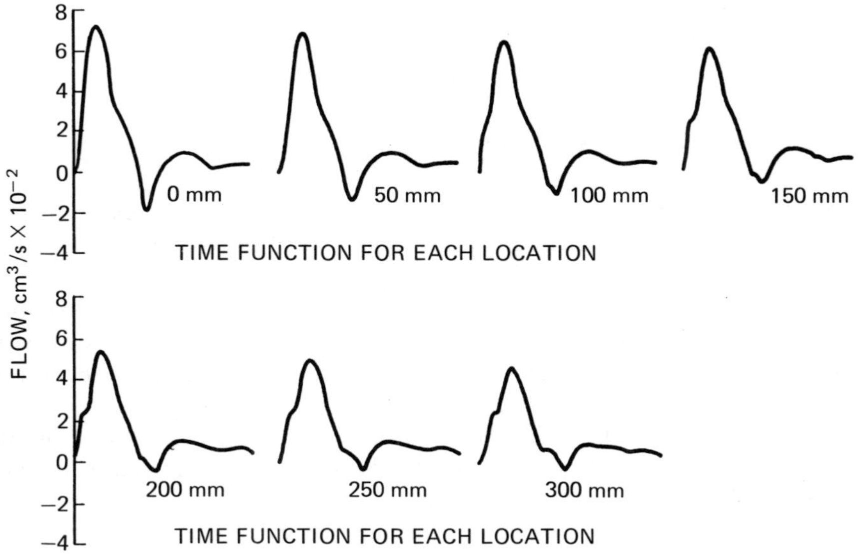

Figure 3–9 Calculated Flow Waveforms along the Aorta.

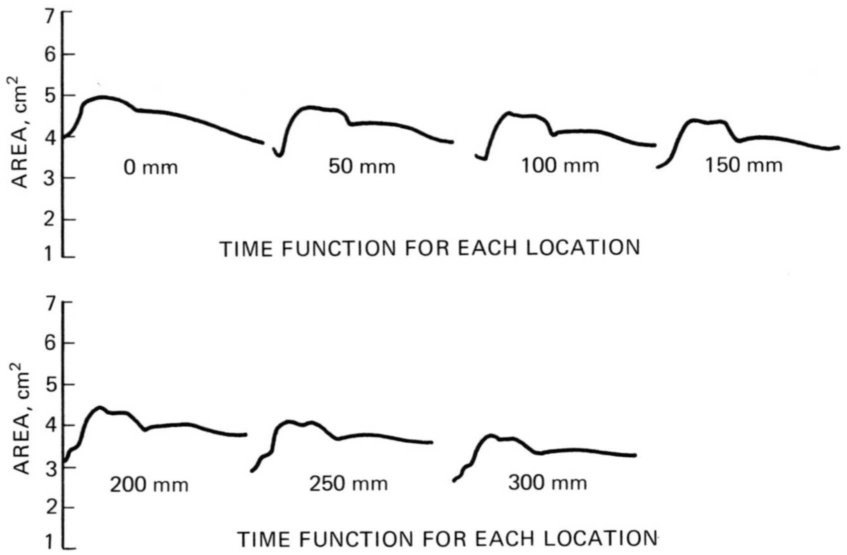

Figure 3–10 Calculated Cross-sectional Area Variations along the Aorta.

It appears, therefore, that this nonreflective, conically tapered, nonlinear model of the aorta is not unreasonable in terms of its predictions of pressure and flow wave propagation in the aorta.

3.2.2 Nonuniform Hybrid Model

In the investigations of a tapered aorta, much effort has been expended on the studies of the nonuniform hybrid model. A variety of techniques have been utilized to attempt to verify the theoretical predictions. These included comparisons with existing data in the literature, comparisons with external plethysmogram measurements on human subjects, and comparisons with results from a series of canine experiments designed to investigate the utility of this theoretical development.

The initial evaluations were carried out using aorta parameters considered reasonable for human pulsatile blood flow. These parameter values are given in Table 3–2. A comparison of the assumed input pressure wave in the ascending aorta (a typical curve) and the calculated aortic pressure waveform at 30 cm, obtained by using the model transfer functions and the parameters of Table 3–2, is shown in Figure 3–11. Five harmonics were used to synthesize the input pressure waveform. Some calculations carried

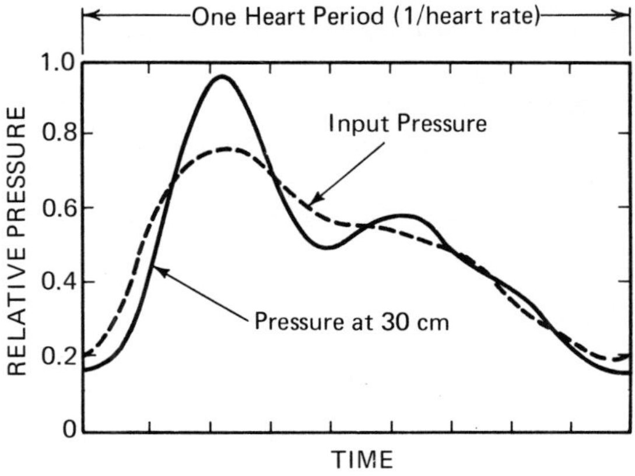

Figure 3–11 Calculated Pressure Waveform for Normal Input (Nonuniform Hybrid Model).

out with 15 harmonics showed no appreciable difference in the time-domain waveform. The calculated output waveform shows the typical rise in systolic peak value, the increase in the dichrotic notch, and the growth of the dichrotic wave (Welkowitz and Fich 1967).

The amplitude and phase characteristics of the input impedance of the hybrid model are shown in Figures 3–5 and 3–6. These are in good agreement with some experimental results taken on a variety of systemic arteries and presented by McDonald (1964).

By utilizing the calculated input impedance function and the assumed input pressure waveform of Figure 3–11, the input flow waveform was calculated and is shown in Figure 3–12. This calculated waveform is in excellent agreement with measured values presented by McDonald (1960).

Table 3–2
Physical Parameters for Initial Verification of Nonuniform Hybrid Model

Parameter, Unit	*Value*
Blood density, kg/m^3	1005
Effective blood viscosity, Ns/m^2	0.04
Heart rate, bpm	75
Ascending aorta, cross-sectional area, m^2	4×10^{-4}
Length of aorta section for calculation, m	0.3
Aorta cross-sectional area at end of section length, m^2	2×10^{-4}
Hoop elasticity (β_e) in ascending aorta, N/m^2	1.6×10^4

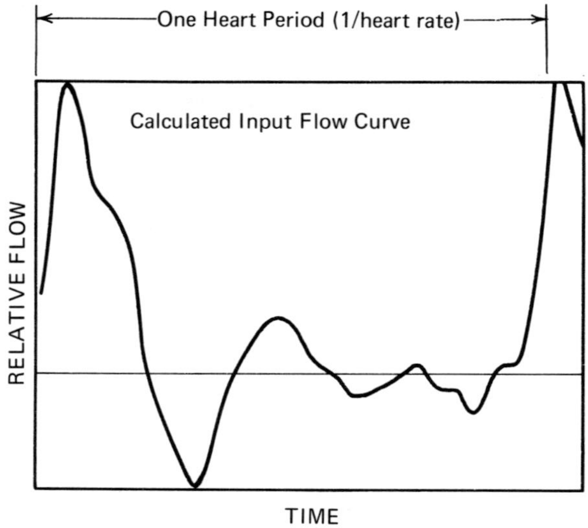

Figure 3–12 Calculated Input Flow Waveform for Normal Pressure Input (Nonuniform Hybrid Model).

Figure 3–11 shows the calculated output pressure waveform for the parameter values of Table 3–2 at a heart rate of 75 bpm. In order to investigate the effects on the pressure of heart rate, similar output pressure waveforms were calculated for heart rates of 131 and 53 bpm, and these are shown in figure 3–13. These results were verified by comparing them with some digital plethysmogram waveforms measured on adult male subjects (Welkowitz and Fich 1967). Digital plethysmograms, which record the displacement of the finger tip under the action of the pressure pulse, produce waveforms similar in shape to the blood pressure pulse. In addition, since the peripheral vascular system consists of small-diameter vessels which are highly resistive, the digital pulse waveform often is quite similar to the waveform in the aorta. Typical digital plethysmogram waveforms measured at high, medium, and low heart rates (120, 80, and 58 bpm) are shown in Figure 3–14. The similarity of the waveform dependence on heart rate illustrated in Figures 3–13 and 3–14 is quite marked. This result suggests that the calculated frequency sensitivity of the pressure wave propagation agrees well with the physiological reality.

The preliminary verifications that have been described thus far led to the design of a series of animal experiments to directly verify the predictions of the nonuniform hybrid aorta model with regard to pressure and flow wave propagation over a wide range of heart rates. Measurements of

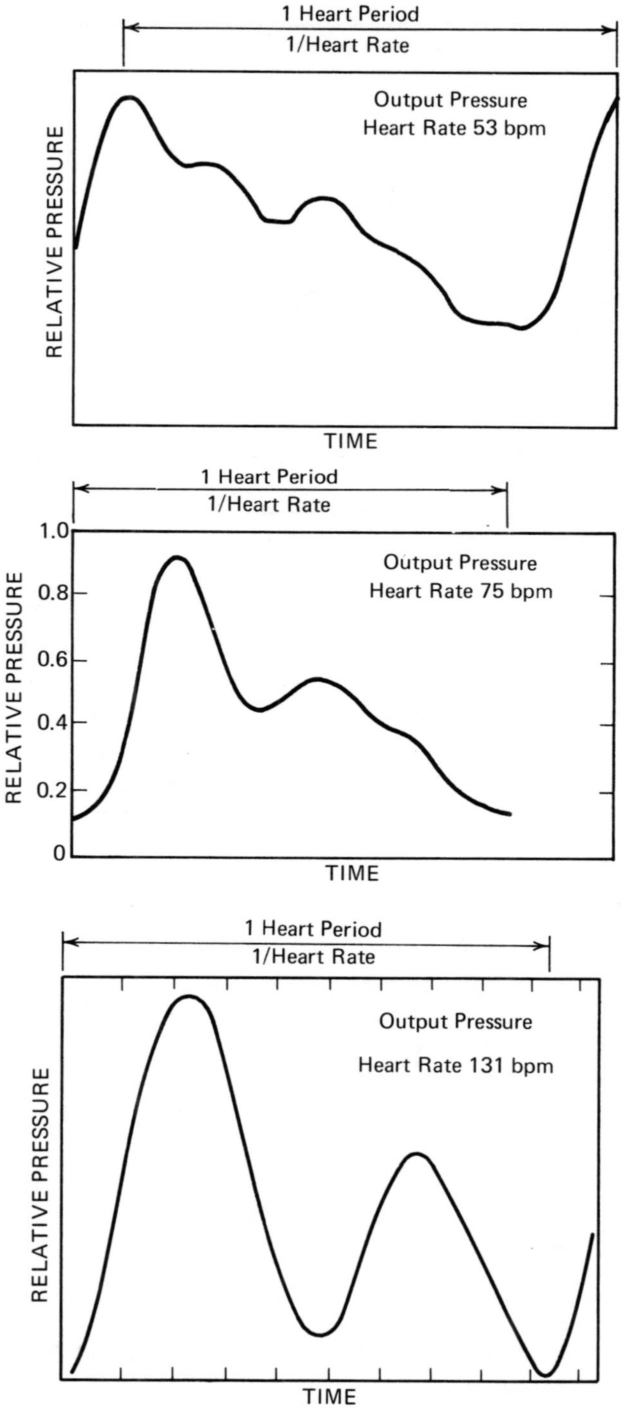

Figure 3–13 Effects of Varying Heart Rate on Calculated Output Pressure Waveforms.

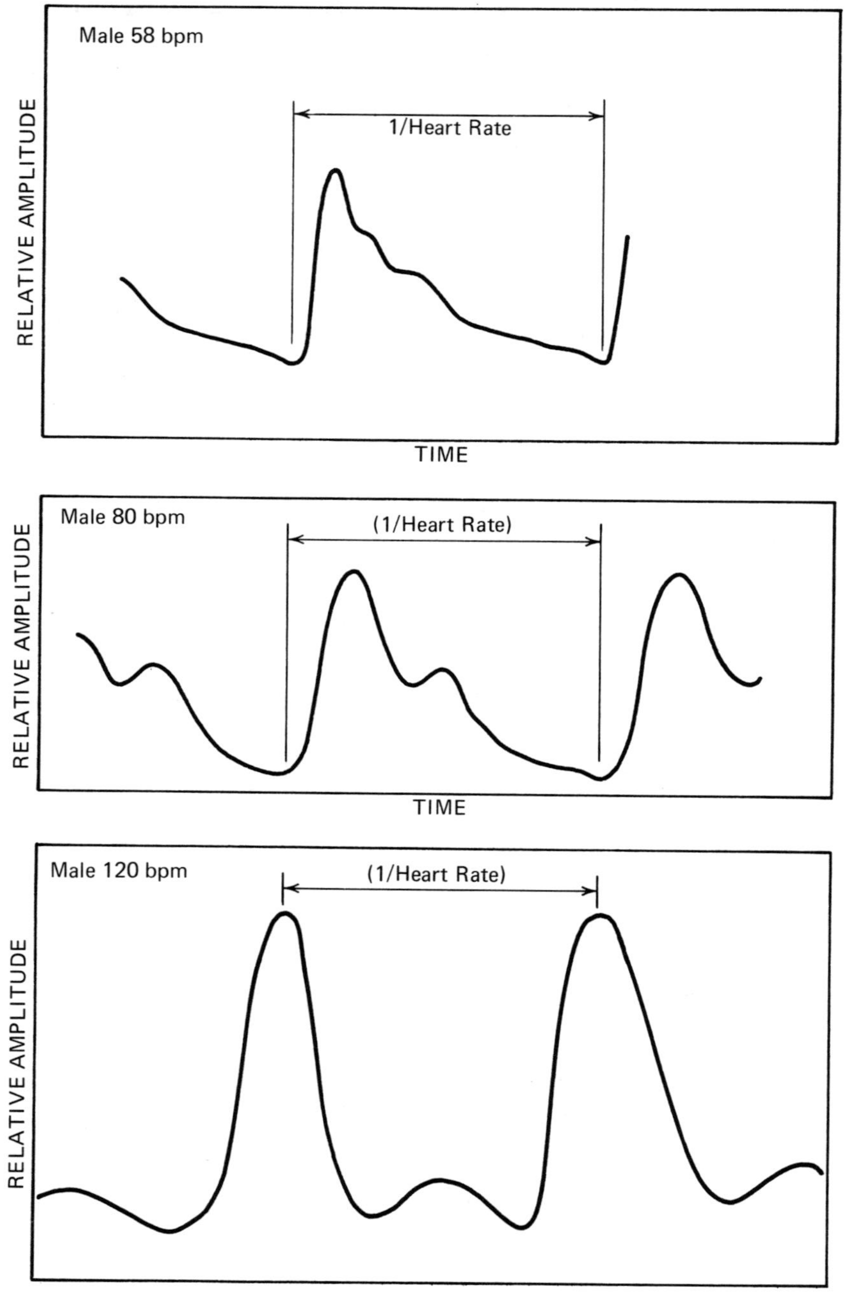

Figure 3–14 Effects of Varying Heart Rate on Measured Digital Plethysmogram Waveforms.

aortic pressure and aortic flow were carried out during *in vivo* experiments on dogs. The measured data have the form of pressure-time curves and flow-time curves recorded on paper-strip charts (Fich et al. 1970).

Dogs were anesthetized intravenously with sodium pentobarbital (30 mg per kg of body weight) and were maintained on an artificial respirator. For the pressure measurements, a polyethylene catheter was inserted through the carotid artery of each dog and was positioned so that the blood pressure near the root of the aorta was measured. One of the femoral arteries was exposed, and another catheter was inserted through the femoral artery into various positions in the thoracic and abdominal aorta. The catheters were filled with saline solution and connected to Statham P23db pressure transducers. Aortic flow was measured using electromagnetic flow probes placed around the aorta. A Biotronex BL610 electromagnetic flowmeter was used for the flow measurements. Zero base line for aortic root flow was assumed to exist during cardiac diastole. A block diagram of this instrumentation including a schematic representation of the aorta showing catheter and flow probe locations is shown in Figure 3–15.

Three types of experiments were carried out in order to provide verification of the hybrid model calculation. In one series of experiments, with the heart rate of the dog kept constant, measurements were carried out with the distal catheter located at various distances (10, 20, and 30 cm) from the proximal catheter so that the functional dependence of the model on distance between transfer function points could be evaluated. In a second series of experiments, the heart rate of the dog was varied by electrical stimulation of the vagus nerve. The catheter positions were kept constant. In this manner, the functional dependence of the model upon heart rate could be verified. In a third series of experiments, distal flow and pressure readings were recorded simultaneously with a proximal pressure reading. The ability of the hybrid model to predict flow functions from pressure measurements could then be evaluated.

In order to utilize the theoretical model for calculating waveforms to be compared with measuremts, various of the physical parameters of the aorta were needed. The nominal values used in these canine studies are shown in Table 3–3. They represent a combination of values obtained from the literature (Patel et al. 1963; Fry, Griggs, and Greenfield 1964) and an evaluation from preliminary experiments.

In all cases, output pressure and flow waveforms were calculated by taking a measured input pressure waveform and multiplying the model transfer function by each harmonic of the input. Then the resultant output harmonics were reconstructed into a time-domain waveform. Ten terms of the Fourier series were used in these calculations. A typical measured input pressure wave complex and its reconstruction from the ten-term series are shown in Figure 3–16. By using these harmonics, output pressure wave-

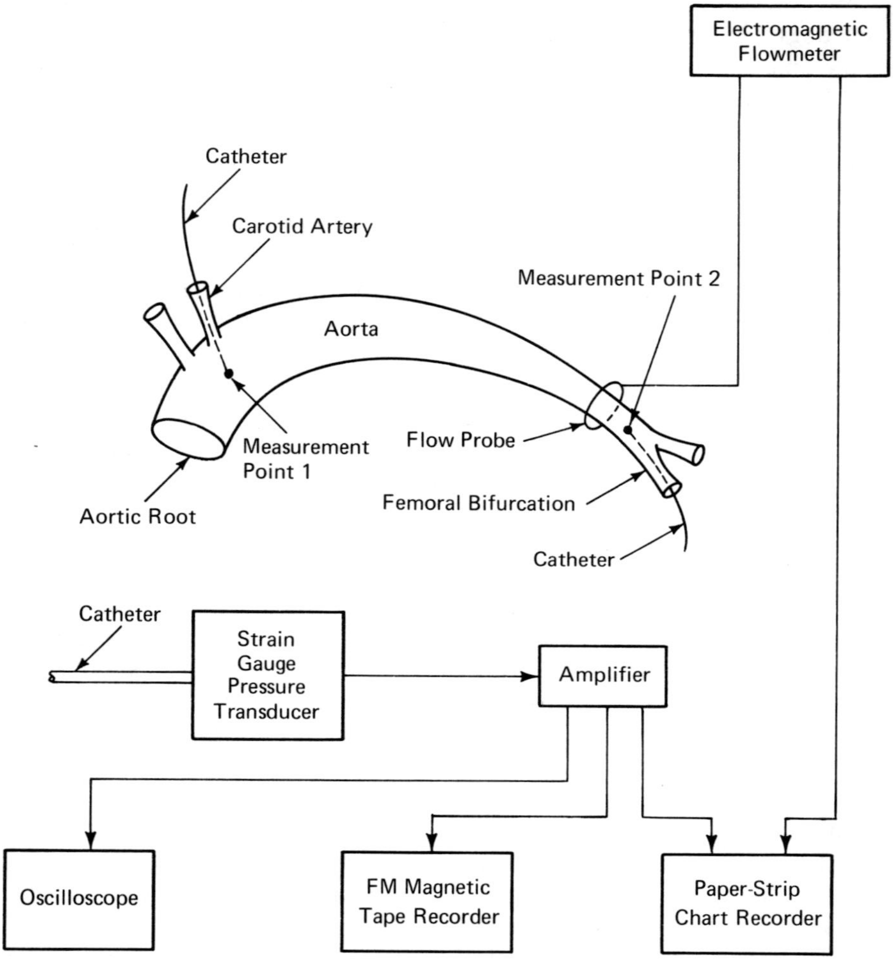

Figure 3–15 Instrumentation for Pressure and Flow Measurements in Dogs.

forms were calculated from the theoretical transfer functions for input-output distances of 10, 20, and 30 cm. Comparisons of the measured pressure waveforms with the calculated pressure waveforms at these locations are shown in Figures 3–17, 3–18, and 3–19. During these measurements the dog's heart rate was maintained at 120 bpm.

With a catheter separation of 20 cm, the heart rate of the dog was varied from 75 to 150 bpm, and pressure measurements were recorded at the

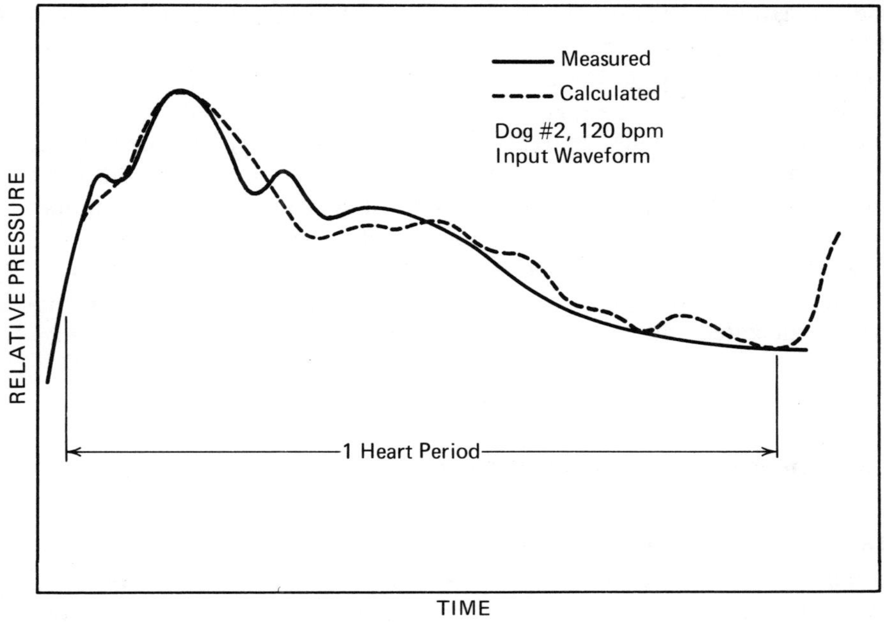

Figure 3–16 Input Pressure Waveform for Model Verification—Measured and Reconstructed Wave.

Table 3–3
Physical Parameters of Canine Studies for Verification of Nonuniform Hybrid Model

Parameter, Unit	*Value*
Blood density, kg/m^3	1004
Effective blood viscosity, Ns/m^2	0.16
Heart rate, bpm	120 fixed
	75–150 variable
Ascending aorta, cross-sectional area, m^2	4×10^{-4}
Length of aorta section for calculation, m	0.1–0.3 variable
	0.2 fixed
	0.415 fixed
Taper constant, m^{-1}	3.5
Hoop elasticity (β_e) in ascending aorta, N/m^2	9.35×10^4
Capacitance in ascending aorta, m^4/N	0.428×10^{-8}

proximal and distal locations. By using the same calculation procedure indicated, output pressure waveforms were calculated for heart rates of 75, 120, and 150 bpm. Comparisons of measured and calculated waveforms for these heart rates are shown in Figures 3–20, 3–21, and 3–22.

In another series of experiments, pressure was measured at the aortic root, and both pressure and flow were simultaneously recorded in the abdominal aorta proximal to the femoral bifurcation. Again, the same calculation technique as has been described was used to predict output waveforms. Comparisons of typical measured and calculated pressure and flow waveforms at the bifurcation are shown in Figures 3–23 and 3–24.

In this extensive group of experiments the reasonable agreement between calculated and measured pressure and flow waveforms is apparent.

3.3 Determination of Aorta Parameters

The good agreement obtained in verification experiments related to the nonuniform hybrid aorta model suggests the possibility that this model can be used in conjunction with simple measurements to determine various physical parameters of the aorta. This determination, if sensitive enough, may have clinical applications.

The procedure for carrying out the determination of aorta parameters that appears reasonable is as follows: if one experimentally measures a steady-state pressure transfer function in the aorta and relates it to the steady-state pressure transfer function of the model, it is possible to adjust the values of the physical parameters that appear in the model until the transfer functions approximately coincide. When this agreement is obtained, it can be assumed that the physical parameters of the model are the phyyical parameters of the aorta (Welkowitz, Fich, and Strano 1972).

If the nonuniform hybrid model of the aorta is accepted as a reasonable representation of the pressure transfer function of the aorta, the crux of the problem is to derive an algorithm by means of which the values of the physical parameters of the aorta are perturbed in a systematic fashion to find the best fit of the magnitude and phase of the transfer functions (Strano 1969; Strano, Welkowitz, and Fich 1972). In this application, the *best fit* is defined as that fit which minimizes the weighted error cost function of Eq. (3–56) which is derived from the measured and calculated transfer functions.

$$y = \sum_{i=1}^{n} [W_{ia}(|t_{pi}| - |g_i|)^2 + W_{ip}(\theta_{ti} - \theta_{gi})^2] \qquad (3\text{–}56)$$

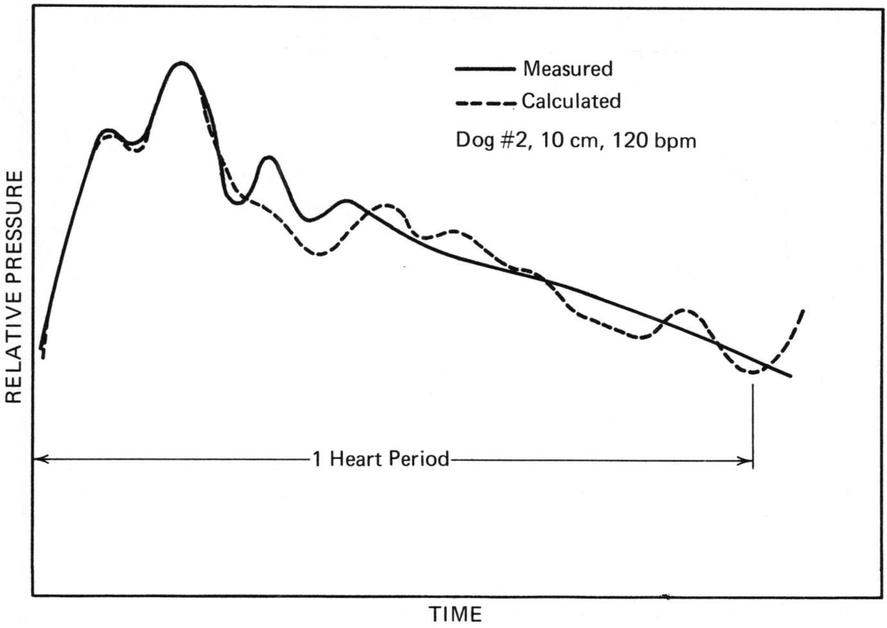

Figure 3–17 Calculated and Measured Pressure Waveforms along the Aorta, 10 cm.

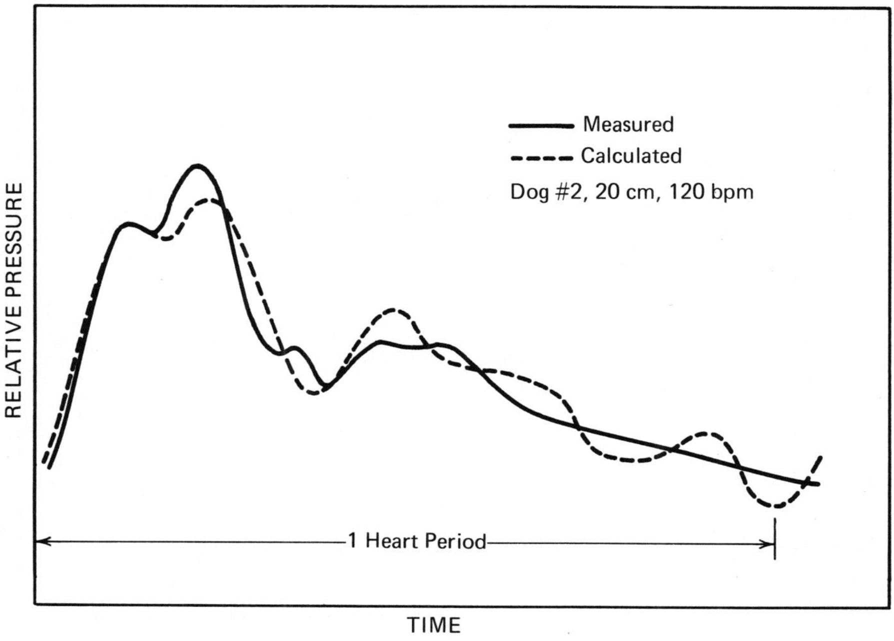

Figure 3–18 Calculated and Measured Pressure Waveforms along the Aorta, 20 cm.

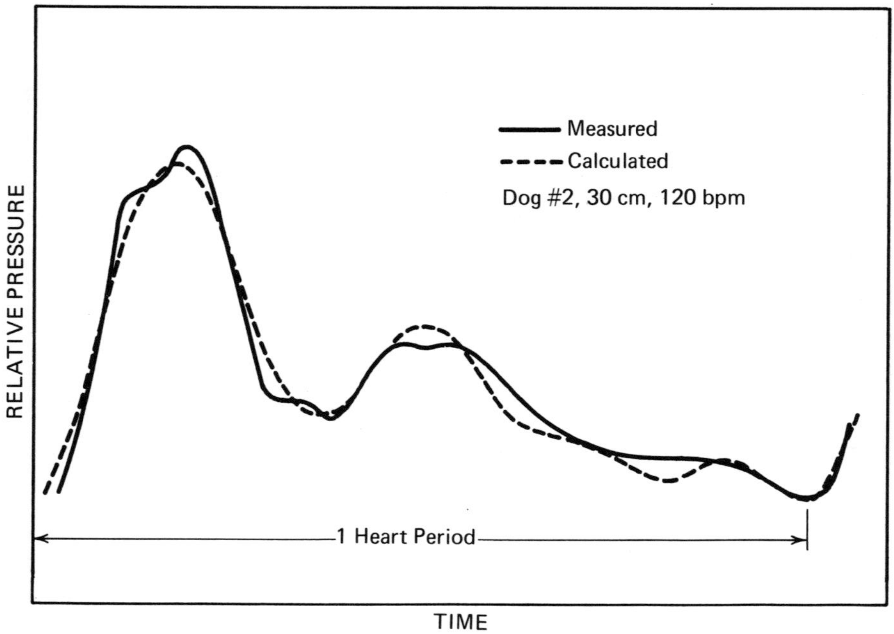

Figure 3–19 Calculated and Measured Pressure Waveforms along the Aorta, 30 cm.

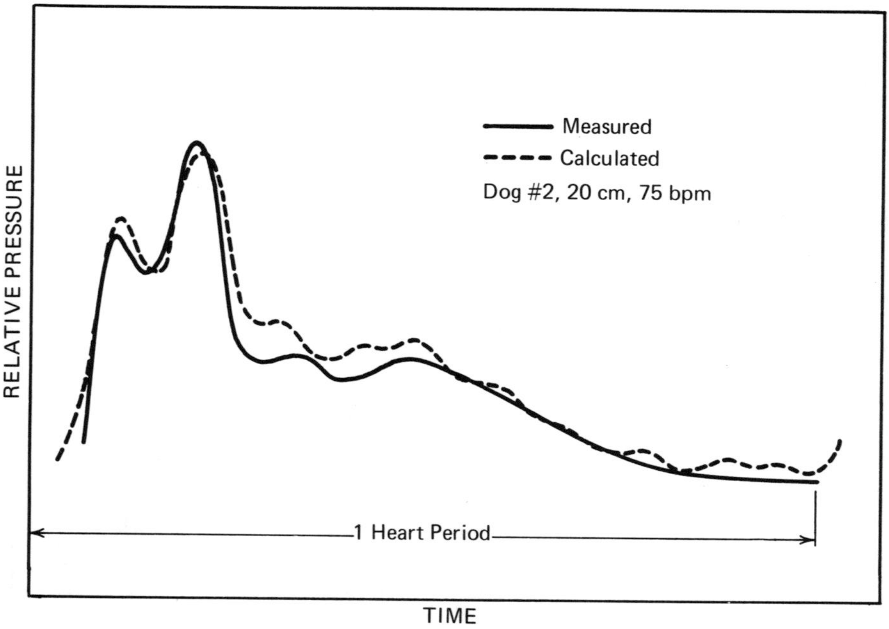

Figure 3–20 Calculated and Measured Pressure Waveforms for Various Heart Rates, 75 bpm.

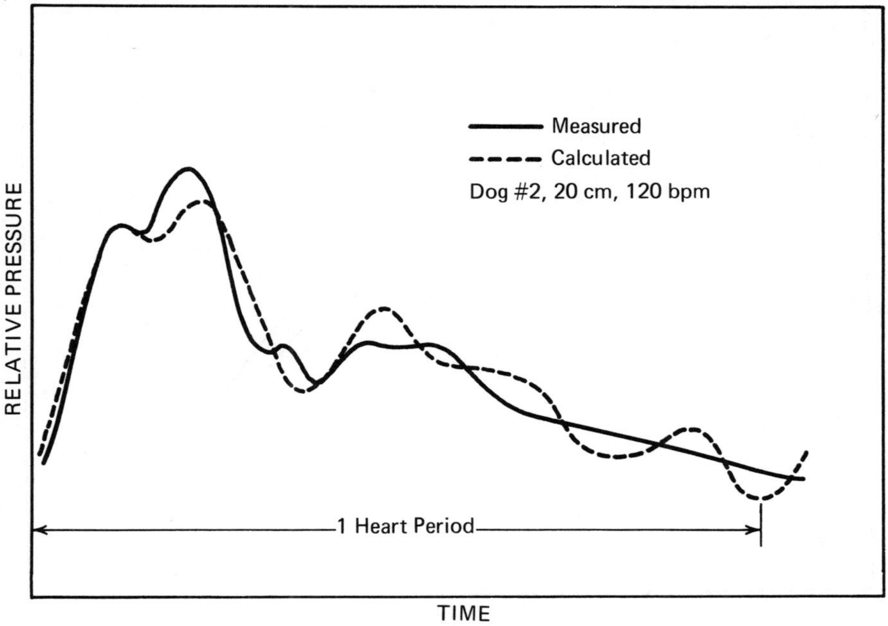

Figure 3–21 Calculated and Measured Pressure Waveforms for Various Heart Rates, 120 bpm.

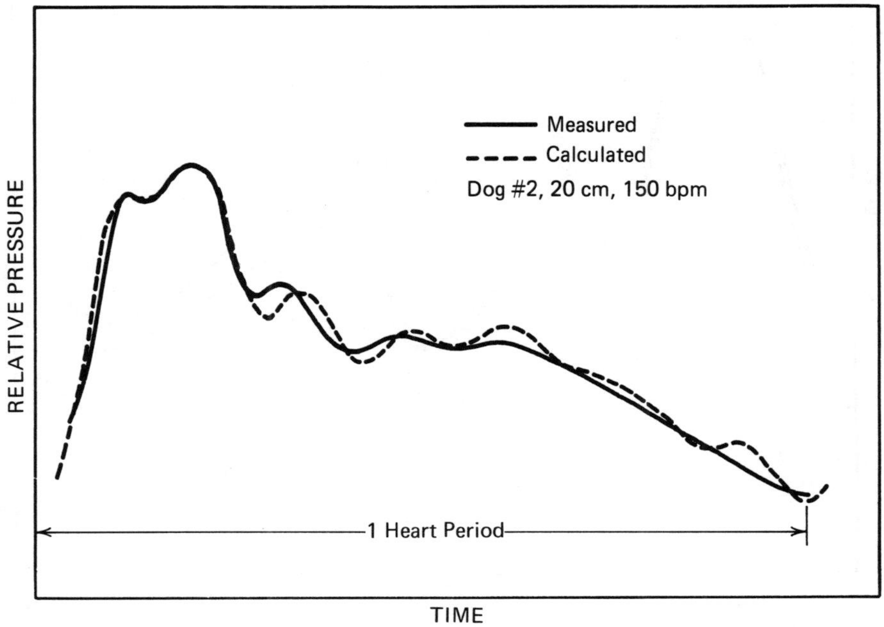

Figure 3–22 Calculated and Measured Pressure Waveforms for Various Heart Rates, 150 bpm.

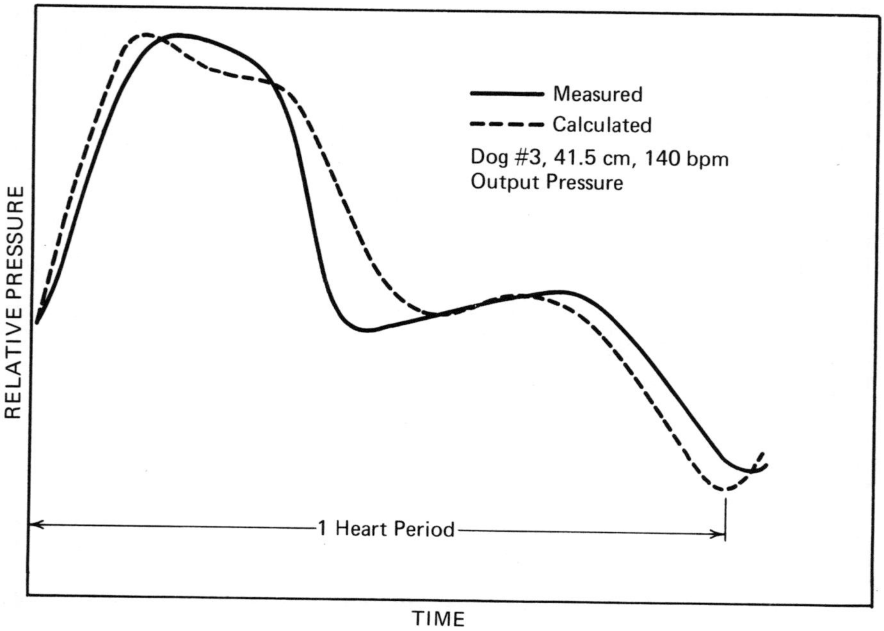

Figure 3–23 Calculated and Measured Pressure Waveforms at Femoral Bifurcation.

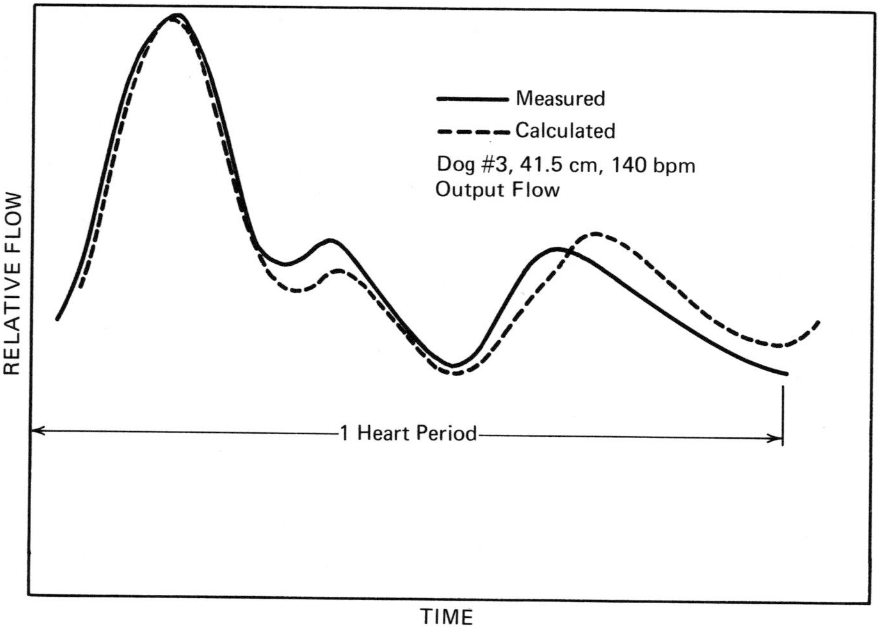

Figure 3–24 Calculated and Measured Flow Waveforms at Femoral Bifurcation.

Table 3–4
Weighting Factors

Frequency	*Amplitude Weighting Factor*	*Phase Weighting Factor*
f_1	1.0	1.0
$2f_1$	0.9	0.9
$3f_1$	0.8	0.8
$4f_1$	0.5	0.1
$5f_1$	0.5	0.1
$6f_1$	0.1	0.0
$7f_1$	0.1	0.0
$8f_1$	0.1	0.0
$9f_1$	0.0	0.0
$10f_1$	0.0	0.0

where y = $y(f_1, f_2, \ldots, R_{a1}, C_{a1}, k, L_a)$, the error measure to be minimized

f_1 = fundamental heart rate ($f_2, \ldots, f_n$ are harmonics of f_1)

n = number of frequency terms used in the harmonic analysis

R_{a1} = hydraulic resistance per unit length at the proximal measurement location

C_{a1} = hydraulic capacitance per unit length at the proximal measurement location

k = taper coefficient of the aorta section between measurement locations

L_a = inertance of the blood in the aorta section between measurement locations

t_{pi} = $|t_{pi}|e^{j\theta_{ti}}$ is the measured pressure transfer function at the ith frequency

g_i = $|g_i|e^{j\theta_{gi}}$ is the model pressure transfer function at the ith frequency

e = $|t_{pi}| - |g_i|$ is the amplitude error of the ith frequency

e_θ = $\theta_{ti} - \theta_{gi}$ is the phase error of the ith frequency

W_{ia} = the weighting factor of the amplitude error

W_{ip} = the weighting factor of the phase error

The choice of the weighting factors can be based upon the relative confidence levels assigned to the measurements of transfer function amplitude and phase at each harmonic of the fundamental heart frequency. In the studies on dogs and chickens to be discussed, the weighting factors shown in Table 3–4 were utilized.

The transfer function of the tapered hybrid model can be obtained from Eqs. (3–43) and (3–47) and is given in Eq. (3–57) in terms of the Laplace transform operator.

$$\frac{P_1(s)}{P_2(s)} = F_1(\gamma l_a) + F_2(\gamma l_a) + F_3(\gamma l_a) + F_4(\gamma l_a) + F_5(\gamma l_a) + F_6(\gamma l_a) \tag{3–57}$$

where

$$F_1(\gamma l_a) = e^{-2kl_a}[\cosh \gamma l_a + (k/\gamma)\sinh \gamma l_a]^2 \tag{3–58}$$

$$F_2(\gamma l_a) = (sR_{a2}C_{a2}/\gamma^2)\left(e^{-2kl_a}\sinh^2 \gamma l_a\right) \tag{3–59}$$

$$F_3(\gamma l_a) = \frac{s^2 l_a C_{a2}}{\gamma}\left[e^{-2kl_a}\sinh \gamma l_a\left(\cosh \gamma l_a - \frac{k}{\gamma}\sinh \gamma l_a\right)\right] \tag{3–60}$$

$$F_4(\gamma l_a) = \frac{\gamma - k}{\gamma^2}\left[e^{-2kl_a}\sinh \gamma l_a\left(\cosh \gamma l_a + \frac{k}{\gamma}\sinh \gamma l_a\right)\right] \tag{3–61}$$

$$F_5(\gamma l_a) = \frac{\gamma - k}{\gamma^2}e^{-2kl_a}\sinh \gamma l_a(\cosh \gamma l_a - k \sinh \gamma l_a) \tag{3–62}$$

$$F_6(\gamma l_a) = \frac{sL_a(\gamma - k)e^{-2kl_a}}{\gamma R_{a2}}(\cosh \gamma l_a + k \sinh \gamma l_a)(\gamma \cosh \gamma l_a - k \sinh \gamma l_a) \tag{3–63}$$

In these equations $P_1(s)$ is the pressure at the location proximal to the aortic root, $P_2(s)$ is the pressure at the location distal to the aortic root, and R_{a2} and C_{a2} are the hydraulic resistance and capacitance per unit length at the location distal to the aortic root.

The optimization strategy used to minimize the value of y in Eq. (3–56) contains the decision-making portion of the optimization procedure. The purpose of the optimization strategy is to adjust the system parameters L_a, R_a, C_a, and k in a prescribed manner so that the error function is minimized in a region of hyperspace. As indicated, four parameters must be simultaneously adjusted to arrive at the minimum error function. In practice, it has been found that a very great amount of computer time is required for the four-parameter optimization. If an approximately correct value of L_a is chosen initially and a three-parameter (R_a, C_a, k) optimization is used, the computer time required is greatly reduced. If necessary, successive approximations to L_a can be chosen to improve the final results. This three-parameter optimization technique was used in the results presented in this chapter.

The steps required to solve the problem iteratively and provide the framework for a computer program are shown in Figure 3–25. A trial parameter set x is chosen and inserted into the model. The model

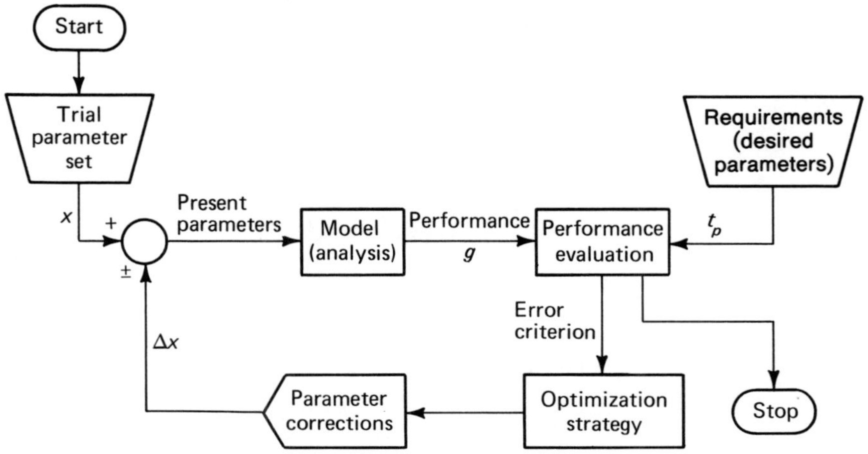

Figure 3–25 Block Diagram of Optimization Procedure.

performance g is computed. The computed values g are compared with the requirements t_p, and the error function is calculated using the chosen criteria. If the performance achieved is within the desired limits of the figure of merit, the calculations stop; otherwise, an optimization algorithm is invoked to produce modifications of the original parameter set. The process is continued until the optimum set of parameters is found or until continued iterations yield negligible improvement (Welkowitz, Fich, and Strano 1972).

The optimization strategy used in a study of this procedure (Strano 1969) to determine the unknown optimum parameters of the model was a combination of well-known techniques such as model reference, elementary learning, modified gradient, and figure of merit methods. A block diagram of the combined optimization technique is shown in Figure 3–26.

The first step in the optimization was to adjust the parameters so that two figures of merit—the frequency and magnitude of the transfer function at its maximum value—were matched. This adjustment provided starting values for the gradient technique. The computer implementation of the modified gradient steepest-descent minimization of the cost function requires the generation of a stepwise gradient vector and a movement given by the negative of this vector direction toward a minimum. In addition, a step size for each direction of the modified gradient must be determined. The details of the steepest-descent procedure and the step size selection, together with flow diagrams and a Fortran program, are discussed by Welkowitz, Fich, and Strano (1972) and Strano (1969).

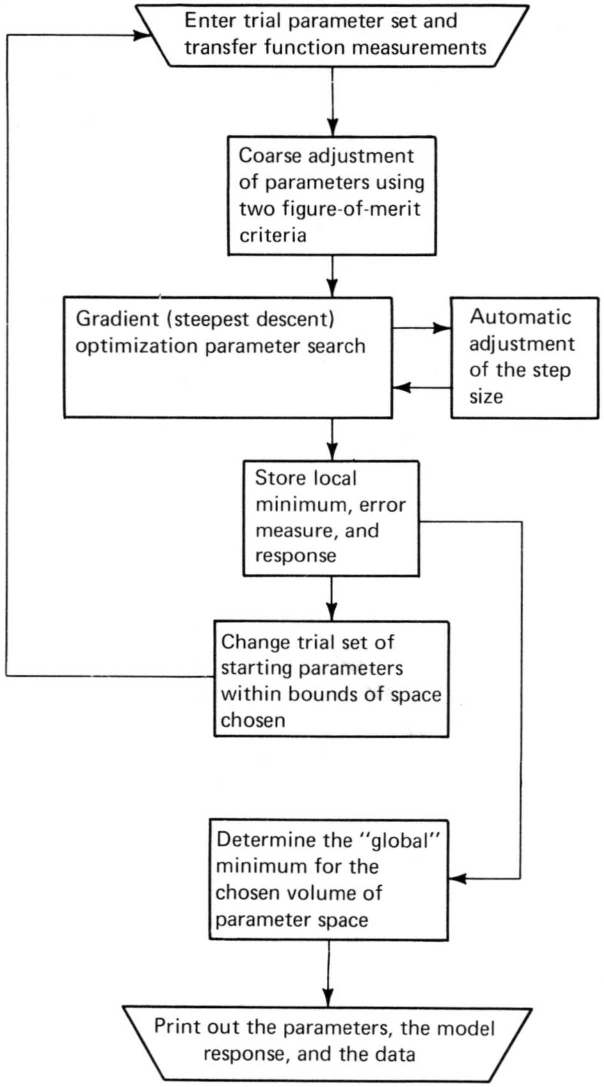

Figure 3–26 Block Diagram of Combined Optimization Method.

The parameter determination program was extensively evaluated using computer-generated test data. In this procedure a table of transfer function "data" was generated by calculation using the model transfer function and preselected values of L_a, R_a, C_a, and k. This set of data was then used as

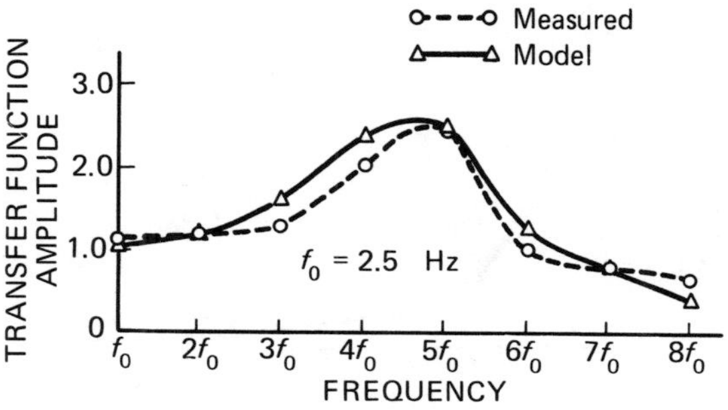

Figure 3–27 Transfer Function Amplitude versus Frequency for Dog Aorta.

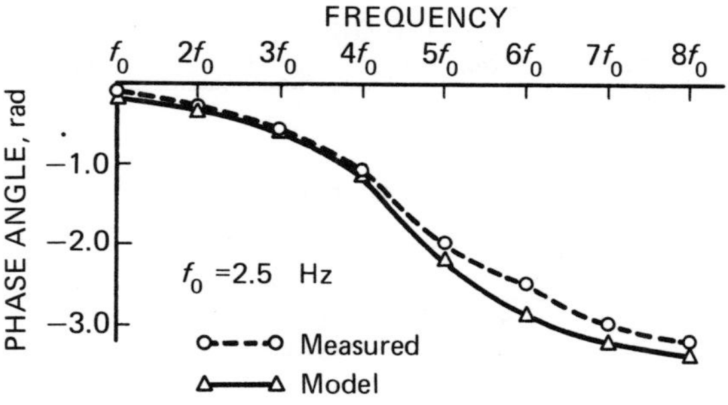

Figure 3–28 Transfer Function Phase Angle versus Frequency for Dog Aorta.

the set of measured values of the transfer function read into the parameter determination program. The algorithm testing procedure consisted of using 164 combinations of trial parameters as initial guesses and allowing the computer program to determine optimum parameters. The initial guesses had a range of ±1000 percent around the original values. In all cases the optimization algorithm converged to the set of preselected values of L_a, R_a, C_a, and k. This numerical testing strongly suggests that the "determination of parameters" procedure is unique.

After pretesting with the concocted "data," the technique was used to determine aorta parameters from actual measurements of transfer functions taken on dogs and chickens. A comparison of measured and model transfer functions is presented in Figures 3–27 to 3–30. These figures show the match between the measured transfer functions and the calculated model

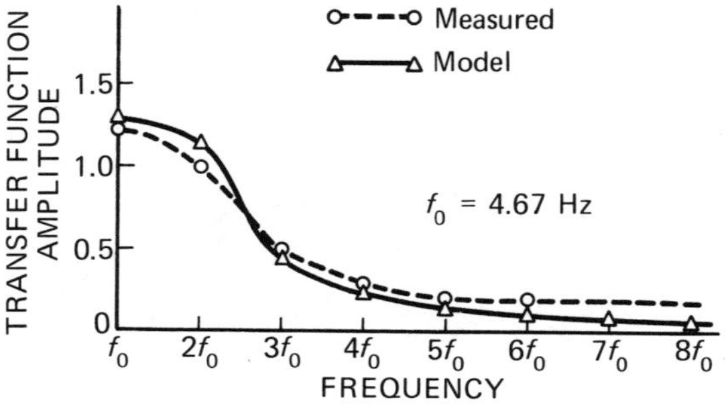

Figure 3–29 Transfer Function Amplitude versus Frequency for Chicken Aorta.

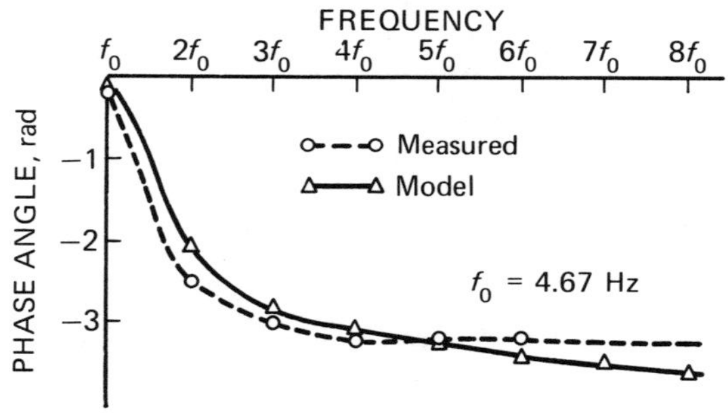

Figure 3–30 Transfer Function Phase Angle versus Frequency for Chicken Aorta.

transfer functions using the computer-derived optimal set of model parameters (Strano, Welkowitz, and Fich 1972). The measured transfer function data were obtained by averaging 40 waveform complexes.

The network parameters R_a, C_a, and L_a are related to physical parameters of the aorta through the definitions following Eqs. (3–9) and (3–10). The taper parameter k is a physical parameter. By using these definitions and the values of R_{a1}, C_{a1}, L_a, and k determined by the optimization algorithm, calculations were carried out of physical parameters for dog and chicken aortas. These results are summarized in Table 3–5 (Strano, Welkowitz, and Fich 1972) together with comparative values from the pertinent literature. It appears that the optimization procedure can yield reasonable values of aorta parameters from simple two-pressure measurements.

Table 3–5
Calculated Aorta Parameters

	Dog		Chicken	
Parameter, Unit	*Calculated Value*	*Literature Value*	*Calculated Value*	*Literature Value*
Taper constant, m^{-1}	4.2	4.72[a]	6.6	7.9[c]
Ascending aorta area, m^2	3.52×10^{-4}	3.81×10^{-4} [a]	0.217×10^{-4}	0.2×10^{-4} [d]
Ascending aorta hoop elasticity, N/m^2	9.0×10^4	3.92×10^4 [a]	1.29×10^4	0.5×10^4 [e] (turkey)
Effective blood viscosity, Ns/m^2	0.24	0.04–0.16[b]	0.225	—

[a] Patel et al. (1963).
[b] Fry, Griggs, and Greenfield (1964).
[c] Direct measurement and fitted exponetial curve.
[d] Weiss, Griminger, and Fisher (1964).
[e] Speckmann and Ringer (1964).

Table 3–6
Range of Typical Parameters for Human Aortas
(*43 runs*)

Taper coefficient	$3.41 - 2.34\ m^{-1}$
Input area (ascending aorta)	$8.64 \times 10^{-4} - 5.7 \times 10^{-4}\ m^2$
Hoop elasticity (ascending aorta)	$12 \times 10^4 - 6.7 \times 10^4\ N/m^2$

Since the technique appears reasonable for determining aorta parameters, Strano (1973) applied it to the *in vivo* determination of human aorta parameters. The measurements were obtained using a double-lumen catheter inserted into the aorta during routine diagnostic catheterization studies. The range of values obtained during this preliminary investigation is given in Table 3–6 (Strano 1973).

From the results obtained using dog, chicken, and human aorta measurements, it appears that this technique for the determination of aorta parameters may well have diagnostic applications.

References

Apter, J.T., "Analysis of Some Effects of Aortic Smooth Muscle on *in vivo* Aortic Pressure Curves," *Bull. Math. Biophys.* 27 (1965): 119.

Attinger, E.O.; Anne, A.; and Sugawara, H., "Model of the Peripheral Vascular System," *Proc. 18th Conf. on Eng. in Med. & Biol.* 7 (1965): 81.

Bergel, D.H., "Arterial Viscoelasticity," in E.O. Attinger, *Pulsatile Blood Flow*, McGraw-Hill Book Co., New York, 1964.

Fich, S.; Welkowitz, W.; and Hilton, R., "Pulsatile Blood Flow in the Aorta," in *Biomedical Fluid Mechanics Symposium*, ASME, 1966, pp. 34–44.

Fich, S.; Welkowitz, W.; Shastri, S.; Freed, P.; and Kantrowitz, A., "Verification of Terminating Impedance for Reflectionless Flow in the Aorta," *Proc. 7th Rocky Mt. Bioengineering Symposium* 1970: 34–42.

Fry, D.L.; Griggs, D.M.; and Greenfield, J.C., "In Vivo Studies of Pulsatile Blood Flow: The Relationship of the Pressure Gradient to the Blood Velocity," in E.O. Attinger, *Pulsatile Blood Flow*, McGraw-Hill Book Co., New York, 1964.

Hilton, R.; Fich, S.; and Welkowitz, W., "Digital Computer Techniques for Testing a Tapered Transmission Line Model of the Human Aorta," *Decus Proc.* (1966): 21–33.

Lawton, R.W., "Measurements on the Elasticity and Damping of Isolated Aortic Strips of the Dog," *Circ. Res.* 3 (1955): 403–408.

McDonald, D.A., *Blood Flow in Arteries*, Edward Arnold Ltd., London, 1960.

———, "Frequency Dependence of Vascular Impedance," in E.O. Attinger, *Pulsatile Blood Flow*, McGraw-Hill Book Co., New York, 1964.

Patel, D.J.; Defreitas, F.M.; Greenfield, J.C.; and Fry, D.L., "Relationship of Radius to Pressure along the Aorta in Living Dogs," *J. Appl. Physiol.* 18 (1963): 1111–17.

———; Greenfield, J.C.; and Fry, D.L., "In Vivo Pressure-Length-Radius Reationship of Certain Blood Vessels in Man and Dog," in E.O. Attinger, *Pulsatile Blood Flow*, McGraw-Hill Book Co., New York, 1964.

Rushmer, R.F., *Cardiovascular Dynamics*, W.B. Saunders Co., Philadelphia, 1961.

Speckmann, E.W., and Ringer, K.K., "Static Elastic Modulus of Turkey Aorta," *Can. J. Physiol. Pharmacol. V.* (1964): 42.

Strano,J.J., "The Application of Learning Model Optimization to the Identification of Distributed Parameters," Ph.D. Thesis, Rutgers University, New Brunswick, N.J., 1969.

———; Welkowitz, W.; and Fich, S., "Measurement and Utilization of in Vivo Blood Pressure Transfer Functions of Dog and Chicken Aortas," *IEEE Trans. Biomed. Eng'g.*, BME-19 (1972): 261–71.

———, "Determination of *in vivo* Human Aorta Parameters," *Proc. 26th ACEMB* (1973): 111.

Streeter, V.L., *Handbook of Fluid Dynamics*, McGraw-Hill Book Co., New York, 1961.

———; Keitzer, W.F.; and Bohr, D.F., "Energy Disipation in Pulsatile Flow through Distensible Taped Vessels," in E.O. Attinger, *Pulsatile Blood Flow*, McGraw-Hill Book Co., New York, 1964.

Talbot, S.A., and Gessner, U., *Systems Physiology*, John Wiley & Sons, New York, 1973.

Taylor, M.G., "Wave Travel in Arteries and the Design of the Cardiovascular System," in E.O. Attinger, *Pulsatile Blood Flow*, McGraw-Hill Book Co., New York 1964.

Watts, R.N., "A Mathematical Model for Studying the Mechanical Properties of the Impaired Left Ventricle," Ph.D. Thesis, Rutgers University, New Brunswick, N.J., 1974.

Weiss, H.S.; Griminger, P.; and Fisher, H., "Correlation between Morphometric Measurements of the Aorta and Visual Scoring of Avion Atherosclerosis," *Anat. Rec.* 148 (4), April 1964.

Welkowitz, W., and Fich, S., "A Nonuniform Hybrid Model of the Aorta," *Trans. N.Y. Acad. of Sci.*, 29 (1967): 316–31.

———; Fich, S.; and Strano, J.J., "Cost Function Analysis Applied to the Determination of Aorta Parameters," *Int. J. Eng'g. Sci.* 10 (1972): 1081–91.

4 Some Models of the Peripheral Vascular System

The models of the aorta that were discussed in Chapter 3 assumed, in the calculations of pressure and flow wave propagation, that the termination at the femoral bifurcation was essentially nonreflective. This concept of reflectionless pulsatile flow in the aorta requires verification (Fich et al. 1970) and some consideration of the characteristics and models of the peripheral vascular system that give rise to this property (Welkowitz 1969).

Three procedures for verifying the reflectionless concept have been explored. The first is based upon a transient experiment in which the heart beat of a dog was stopped by electrical excitation of the vagus nerve, and the transient pressure waveform during recovery is observed. The first recovery waveform, substantially unaffected by reflection, had essentially the same form as the later steady-state pulsatile waveforms. This suggests that phenomena other than reflection from the femoral bifurcation produced the observed waveform modifications. The second procedure has already been extensively considered in Chapter 3. It consists of comparing observed and calculated waveforms when the calculations are derived from the dispersive characteristics of the aorta caused by the geometric and elastic taper with reflection eliminated. By using this technique and nominal values of aorta parameters, calculated waveforms are found to be in good agreement with observed values. The third procedure consists of calculating reflection coefficients at the aorta termination using a measured terminating impedance obtained from observed pressure and flow waveforms. A Fourier analysis is used to determine the frequency components in the pulsatile steady state, and then the impedance components can be calculated. The reflection coefficients are calculated from this measured terminating impedance and a quasi-characteristic impedance of the aorta near the termination obtained from nominal aorta parameters. These calculated reflection coefficients have a maximum value of 14 percent for the fundamental frequency and next two higher harmonics. These three frequencies contain practically all the pulsatile energy.

While these verification experiments suggest that a reasonably good impedance match exists at the femoral bifurcation, they also demonstrate that there is some reflection. In addition, it is well known that the peripheral vascular system is under neural control which changes the diameter (and flow resistance) of the peripheral vessels. Thus, the peripheral hydraulic impedance must vary to some extent. Some of the effects of mismatch at the peripheral termination were analyzed for the nonuniform hybrid aorta model (Welkowitz and Fich 1967), and they are shown in Figures 4–1 and 4–2. It appears from these calculations that a moderate variation of terminal impedance has a minimal effect on the important hemodynamic characteristics such as the pulsatile afterload presented to the heart and the amplitude of the pulse pressure.

A somewhat better understanding of the performance of the peripheral vascular system can be obtained by examining a network equivalent model of the femoral system and by relating this model to such physiological measurements as the femoral artery input impedance, pressure transfer functions along the femoral artery, and the effects of drug-induced dilation and constriction on these measurements. Later in this chapter two network structures which model the vascular peripheral system are investigated—a π network and a split π network. Both show some promise as models of this portion of the vascular system.

4.1 Experimental Verification on Nonreflection

Figure 4–3 shows the pulsatile steady-state and recovery pressure waveforms simultaneously in the ascending and the abdominal aorta in a dog after the heart was stopped by electrical excitation of the vagus nerve. The first recovery waveform, propagated along a substantially quiescent vessel and therefore unaffected by reflection, is observed to have essentially the same shape as the later steady-state waves. This observation holds at both locations along the aorta. It suggests that reflection at the femoral bifurcation has a minimal effect on the wave propagation in the aorta.

As was suggested in the Introduction, an additional approach to verification of nonreflection from the femoral bifurcation consists of the measurements of the impedance at this location and the calculation of appropriate reflection coefficients for the significant harmonics of the waveform. Strano, Welkowitz, and Fich (1972) have shown that only the first three frequencies contain significant amounts of energy. Time-domain waveforms of flow and pressure measured in a dog at the femoral bifurcation are illustrated in Figure 4–4. A Fourier analysis of the measured waveforms yields the pressure, flow, and impedance phasors for each harmonic. These are designated as P_{2m}, Q_{2m}, and Z_{2m} where

$$Z_{2m} = \frac{P_{2m}}{Q_{2m}} \tag{4–1}$$

for each Fourier component.

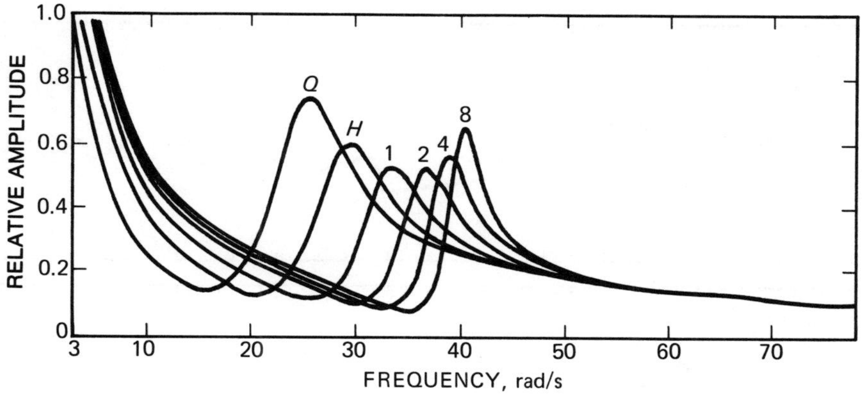

Figure 4–1 Variation of Calculated Input Impedance of Aorta with Varying Terminal Impedance.

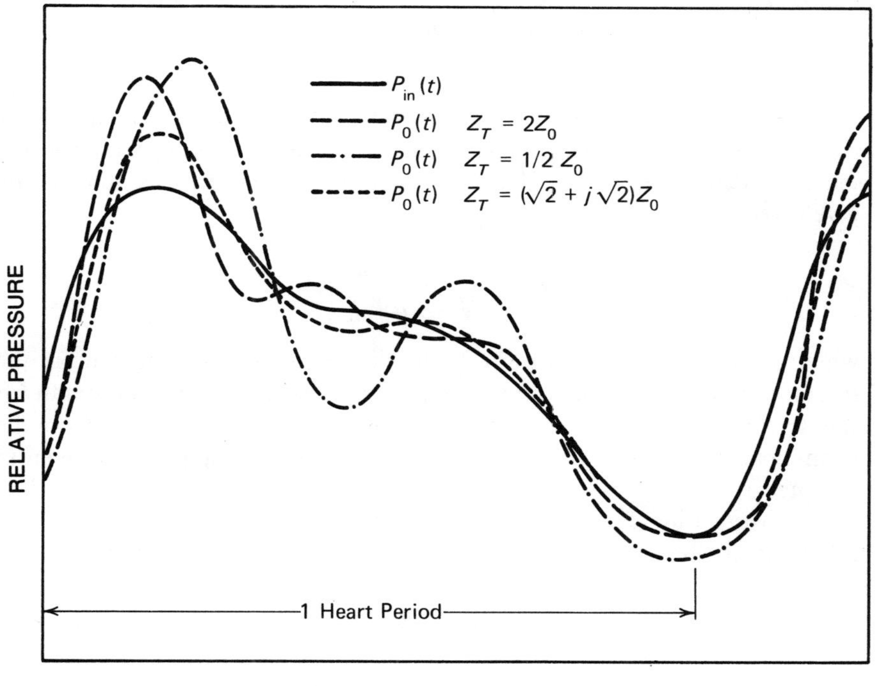

Figure 4–2 Variation of Calculated Output Pressure Waveform with Varying Terminal Impedance.

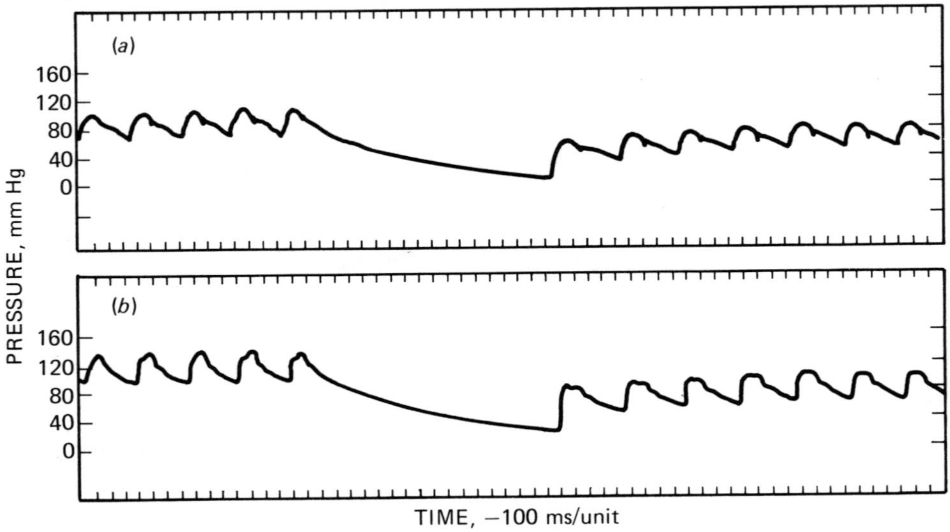

Figure 4–3 Transient and Steady-State Pressure Measurements in the Ascending and Abdominal Aorta.

The reflection coefficients at the bifurcation can be calculated by assuming that the aorta consists of a uniform section just proximal to the measurement location. The characteristic impedance of this section for any given frequency is

$$Z_0 = \sqrt{\frac{R_{a2} + j\omega L_{a2}}{j\omega C_{a2}}} \tag{4–2}$$

where R_{a2}, L_{a2}, and C_{a2} are the hydraulic resistance per unit length, the inertance per unit length, and the hydraulic capacitance per unit length for this section. Nominal values of these parameters can be calculated from the formulas and tables of physical constants of the aorta and blood given in Chapter 3.

By using this characteristic impedance Z_0, the absolute value of the reflection coefficient for any Fourier component of the waveforms is

$$|\rho_r| = \left|\frac{Z_{2m} - Z_0}{Z_{2m} + Z_0}\right| \tag{4–3}$$

Employing the waveforms of Figure 4–4 and the nominal values of aorta parameters, Table 4–1 presents calculations of measured impedance, characteristic impedance, and absolute value of the reflection coefficients for the

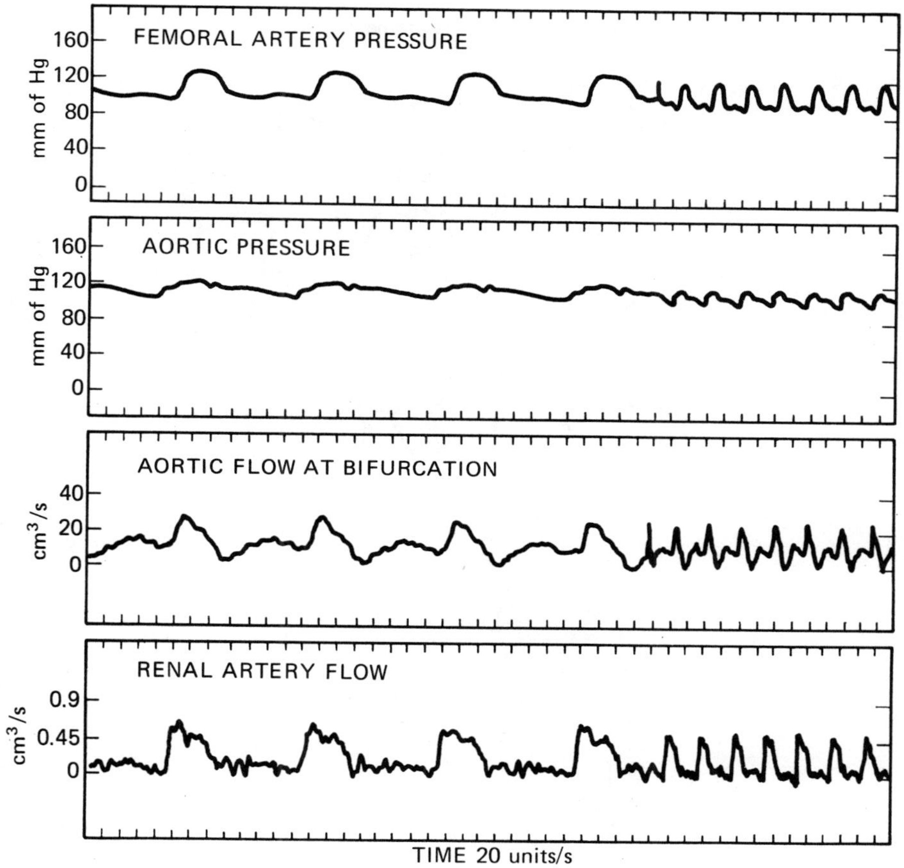

Figure 4–4 Flow and Pressure Waveform Measurements in a Dog at the Femoral Bifurcation.

first three harmonics of the observed waveforms. It can be seen from Table 4–1 that, for this experiment, the reflection coefficients for each of the first three harmonics are practically constant and quite small. These results suggest that reflection at the femoral bifurcation has a minimal effect on wave propagation in the aorta.

4.2 Measurements in Canine Femoral Artery

It is generally necessary, in studying the systemic circulatory system, to know more about the peripheral circulation than just the terminating

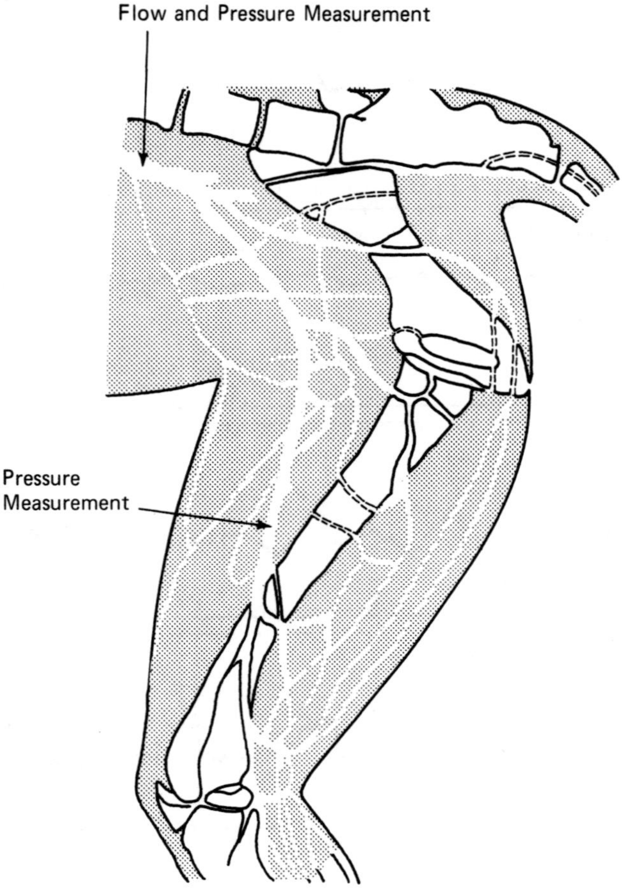

Figure 4–5 Circulatory Anatomy of the Dog's Hind Leg.

Table 4–1
Reflection Coefficients at Femoral Bifurcation

Harmonic	*Measured Impedance*	*Characteristic Impedance*	*Reflection Coefficients*
ω_n	Z_{2m}	Z_0	$\lvert\rho_r\rvert$
$\omega_1 = 5\pi$	$7.6/\underline{-36^\circ}$	$6.2/\underline{-26^\circ}$	0.13
$\omega_2 = 10\pi$	$5.3/\underline{-32^\circ}$	$5.3/\underline{-17^\circ}$	0.13
$\omega_3 = 15\pi$	$4.0/\underline{-20^\circ}$	$5.1/\underline{-12^\circ}$	0.14

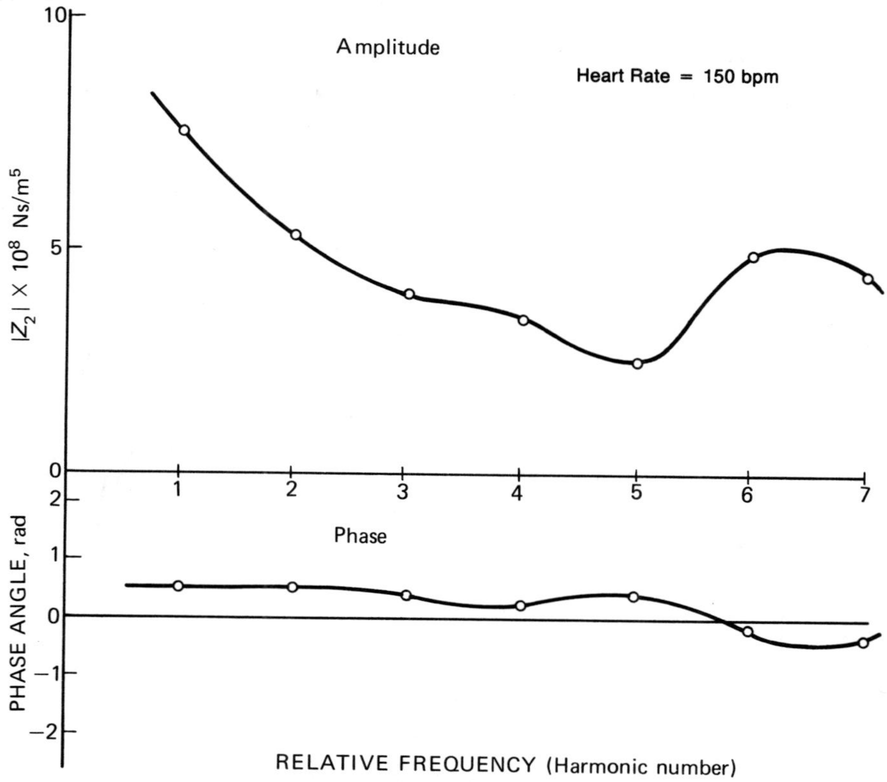

Figure 4–6 Terminating Impedance of the Aorta.

characteristics at the aorta. In a manner similar to that used to study the aorta, an engineering analysis of the femoral artery can be carried out by making measurements of input impedance and transfer functions under a variety of physiological conditions and then attempting to establish mathematical models to explain these measurements.

Measurements were carried out on the femoral artery of a dog (Welkowitz 1969) at the locations shown on the anatomical drawing of Figure 4–5. The input impedance measured at the femoral bifurcation (using pressure and flow measurements) is shown in Figure 4–6. It has the same shape as similar measurements on both dogs and humans presented by McDonald (1964). Pressure transfer function amplitude curves measured at a number of different times are shown in Figure 4–7. Since the cross-sectional area of the capillaries varies with time under neural control, one could expect the observed variations of the magnitude of the pressure transfer function.

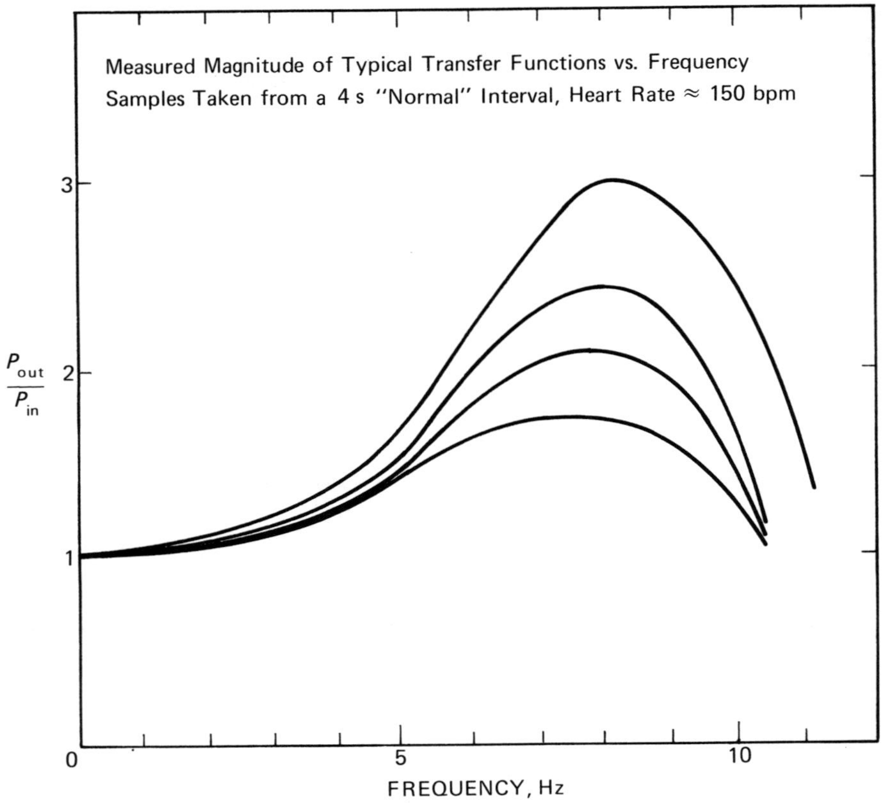

Figure 4–7 Measured Pressure Transfer Function Magnitudes in the Dog's Femoral Artery.

Drug studies of the effect of deliberately varying the diameters of the peripheral vessels using both a dilator drug (Thorazine) and a constrictive drug (Seracaine) were carried out to further elucidate this property of the peripheral vascular system. The effect of Thorazine on the impedance at the femoral bifurcation can be observed by comparing Figure 4–8 with Figure 4–6. The effect of Seracaine on the pressure transfer function amplitude is shown in Figure 4–9.

4.3 Equivalent Network Models

Some preliminary investigations of network models were carried out in order to explain the various experimental results. For the case of the

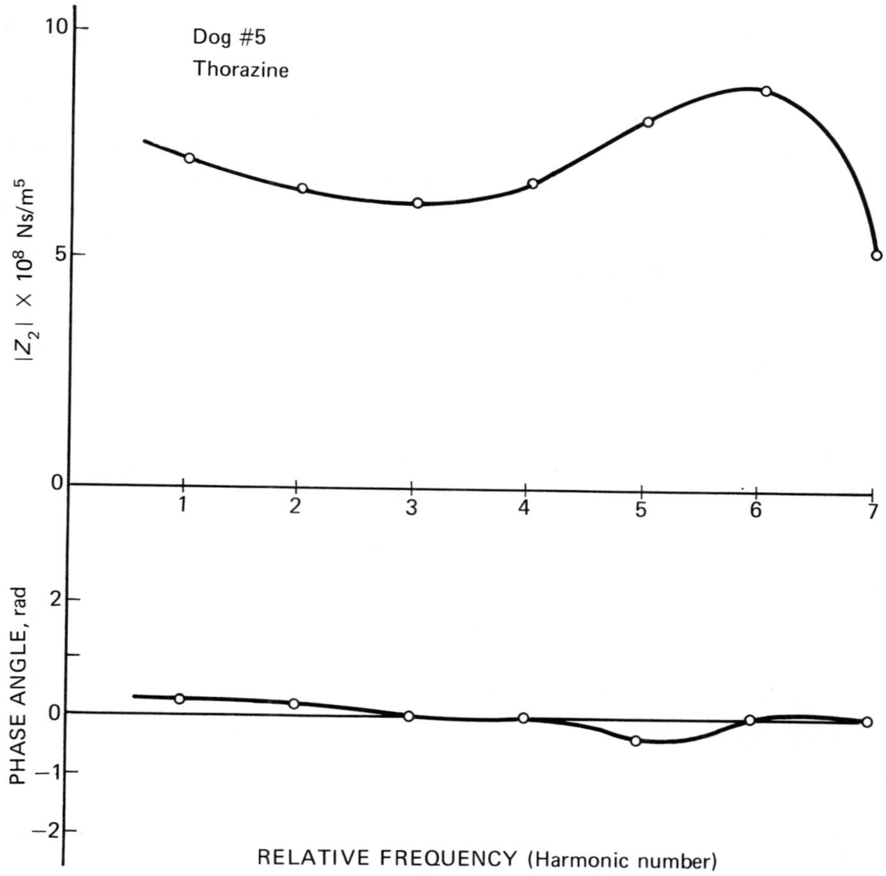

Figure 4–8 Effect of Thorazine on Terminating Impedance of the Aorta.

"normal" dog (no drug excitation, no vagal nerve stimulation) the two-port lumped-parameter π-section network model shown in Figure 4–10 was analyzed. In this model L_f is the inertance of the blood in the femoral artery, R_f is the hydraulic resistance caused by viscous flow effects at the walls, C_f is the hydraulic capacitance produced by the elasticity of the vessel wall, and R_T is the terminal resistance representing viscous loss in the capillaries. Using the parameter definitions given in Chapter 3 and assuming that the femoral artery section being studied is approximately uniform in cross section, it can be expected that the parameters vary functionally with the effective cross-sectional area as follows:

$$L_f = K_1 A^{-1} \tag{4–4}$$

$$R_f = K_2 A^{-2} \tag{4–5}$$

$$C_f = K_3 A^{3/2} \tag{4–6}$$

Nominal values for the parameters of the model were selected by computer analysis to yield a "good fit" of the shape of the model transfer function when compared to the measured femoral artery pressure transfer function. These nominal values are given in Table 4–2. Figure 4–7 illustrates the variations of the pressure transfer function magnitude with the fluctuation of peripheral resistance caused by the neurally controlled variations of capillary cross section. The equivalent effect on the network model transfer function of varying R_T from 10 to 100 Ω is shown on the computer printout of Figure 4–11. This computed effect is quite similar to the physiological variation measured and shown in Figure 4–7.

The computed input impedance functions of the π-section model using the nominal values of Table 4–2, but varying the input capacitance, are shown in Figures 4–12 and 4–13 for the amplitude and phase responses respectively. The experimental points from Figure 4–6 are superimposed for comparison.

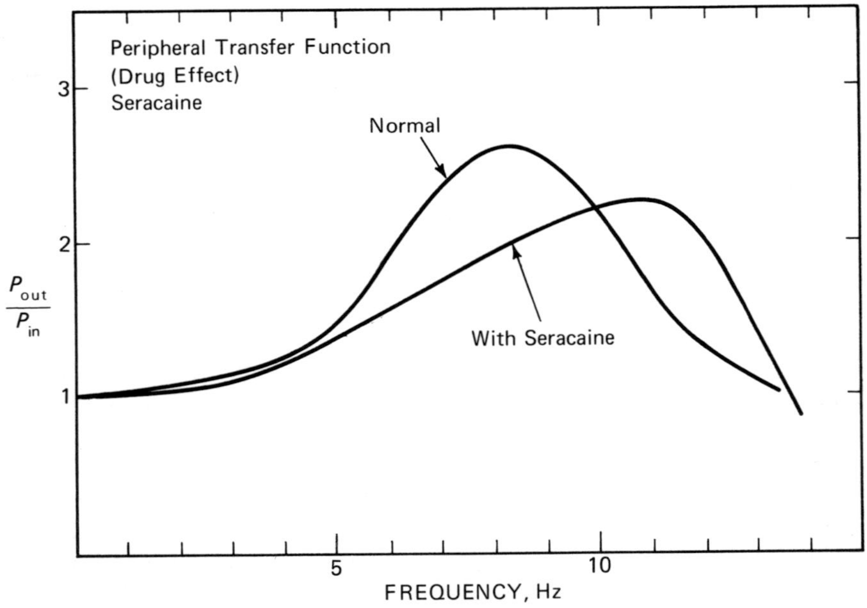

Figure 4–9 Effect of Seracaine on Pressure Transfer Function Magnitude in the Femoral Artery.

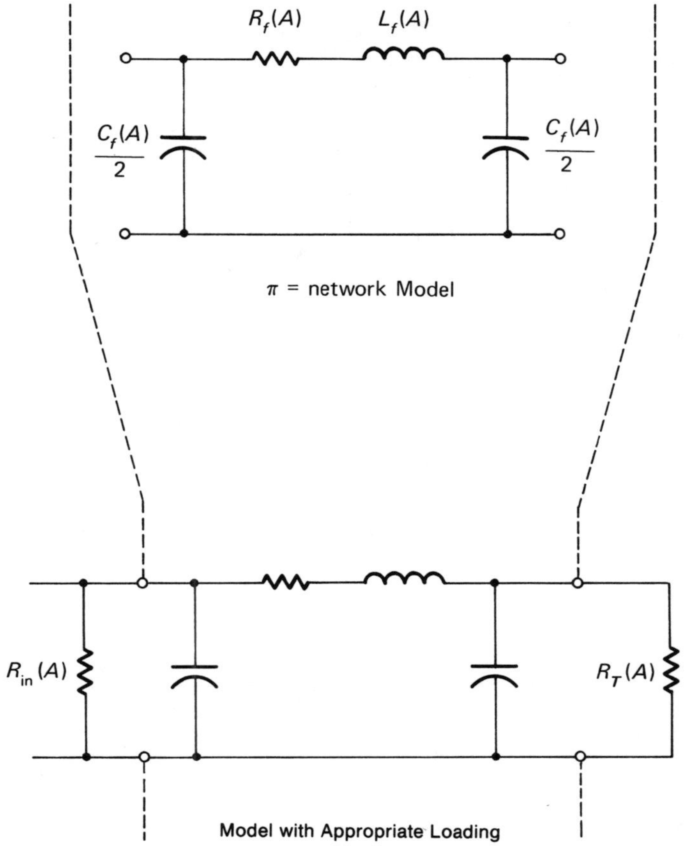

Figure 4–10 Network Models of Femoral Artery.

Table 4–2
Nominal Model Parameters

Parameter	*Network Values*	*Hydraulic Values*
R_f	1.45 Ω	2.18×10^8 Ns/m^5
R_T	35 Ω	52.5×10^8 Ns/m^5
L_f	0.1 H	0.15×10^8 kg/m^4
$C_f/2$	0.004 μ F	2.67×10^{-11} m^5/N

The results shown in Figures 4–11, 4–12, and 4–13 indicate that the π-section network model may be useful in describing the functioning of the femoral artery under normal conditions. This work was followed by an

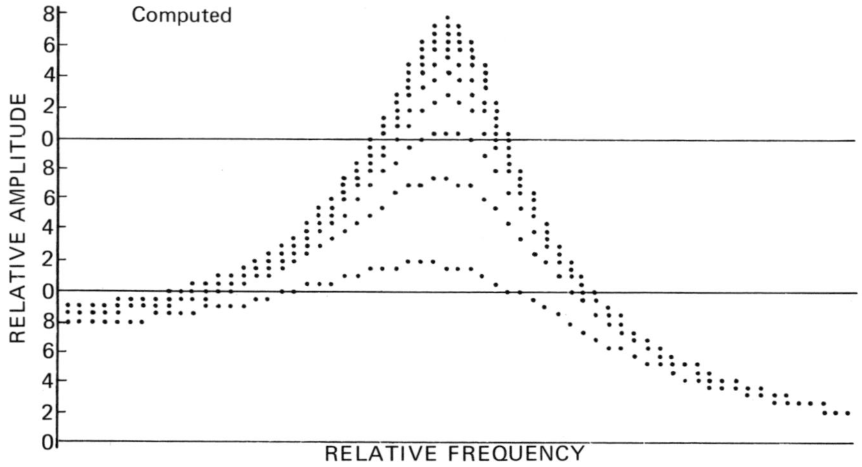

Figure 4–11 Computer Network Model Transfer Function with Varying Load.

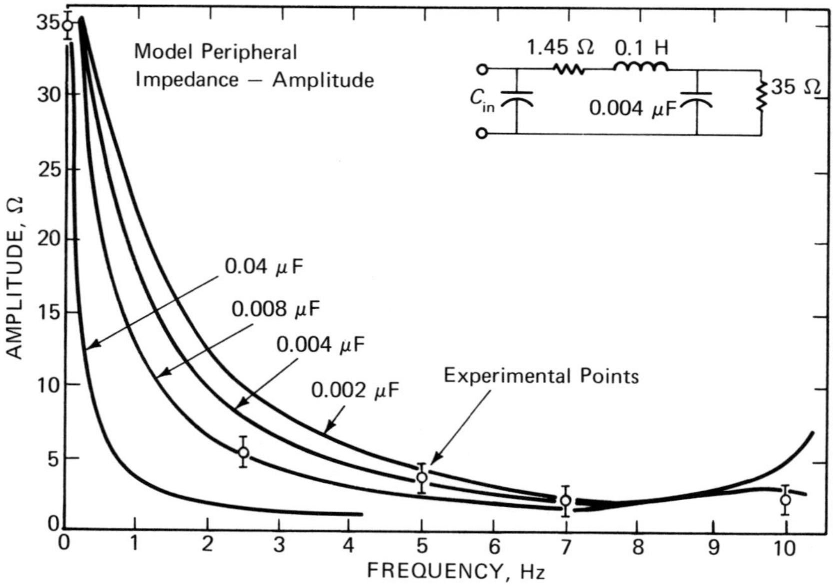

Figure 4–12 Computed Variation of Network Input Impedance Amplitude Function with Varying Input Capacitance.

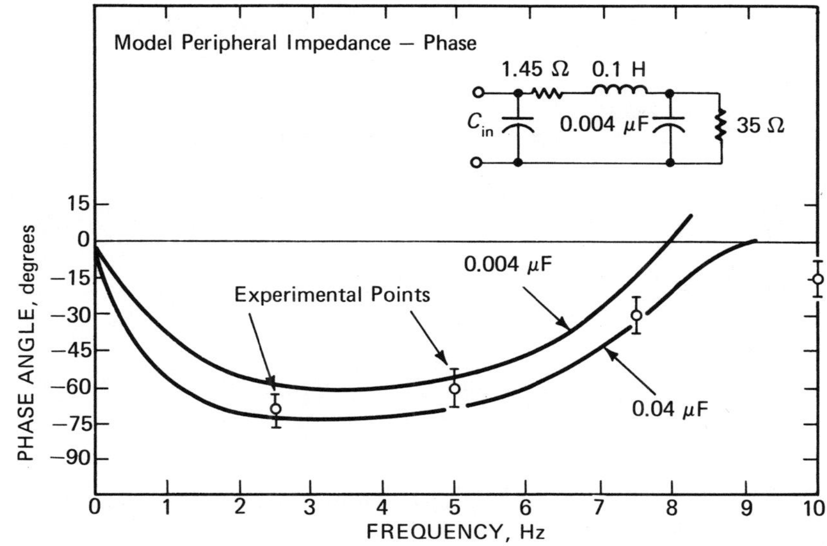

Figure 4–13 Computed Variation of Network Input Impedance Phase Function with Varying Input Capacitance.

investigation into the applicability of the model in explaining the effects of constricting and dilating drugs such as Seracaine and Thorazine. In particular, a detailed analysis was carried out to study the effects of constriction (Seracaine experiments). The experimental effect of Seracaine, as illustrated in Figure 4–9, is to shift the peak of the peripheral transfer function upward in frequency and to reduce Q_M slightly. A computer study of the model of Figure 4–10 indicates that it is not possible to match these results using the area functions of Eqs. (4–4), (4–5), and (4–6) either singly or in groups. However, by splitting the model into a large artery section that is not area-dependent and a small artery section that is area-dependent, agreement can be obtained between the computer calculations based upon the model and the constrictive-drug experiments. This split π model is shown in Figure 4–14 with the nominal circuit element values shown on the diagram. The computed effects of varying the area parameter on the amplitude of the transfer function of the split π network are shown in Figure 4–15. A comparison of these calculations with the Seracaine experiments (Figure 4–9) suggests that Seracaine affects only the distal portions of the femoral artery and the smaller vessels following, but does not affect the proximal portions of this vessel.

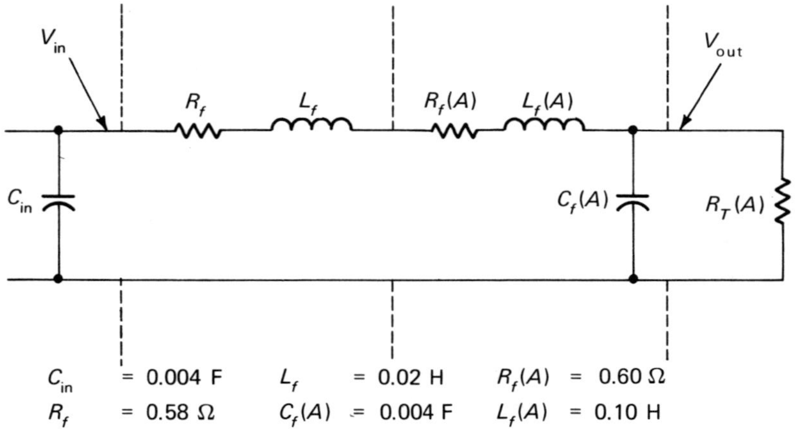

Figure 4–14 Split π Network Model of Femoral Artery (as Suggested by Drug Experiments).

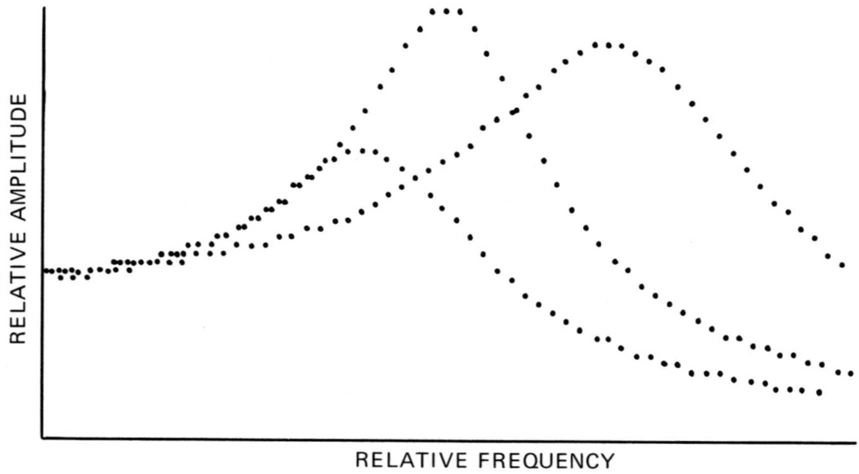

Figure 4–15 Computed Variation of Network Model Transfer Functions with Varying Area.

As indicated, this work on models of the peripheral vascular system is only preliminary. Further studies are needed (as are more elaborate models) to investigate dilation and constriction effects and the effects of heart rate variations. The models investigated thus far have been lumped networks. As in the case of the aorta, distributed networks or hybrid models may be needed. There is a need for much additional research and study of the peripheral vascular system.

References

Fich, S.; Welkowitz, W.; Shastri, S.; Freed, P.; and Kantrowitz, A., "Verification of Terminating Impedance for Reflectionless Flow in the Aorta," *Proc. 7th Rocky Mt. Bioengineering Symposium* (1970): 34–42.

McDonald, D.A., "Frequency Dependence of Vascular Impedance," in E.O. Attinger, *Pulsatile Blood Flow*, McGraw-Hill Book Co., New York, 1964.

Strano, J.J.; Welkowitz, W.; and Fich, S., "Measurement and Utilization of *in Vivo* Blood Pressure Transfer Functions of Dog and Chicken Aortas," *IEEE Trans. Biomed. Eng.* BME-19 (1972): 261–71.

Welkowitz, W., and Fich, S., "A Non-uniform Hybrid Model of the Aorta," *Trans. N.Y. Acad. Sci.* 29 (1967): 316–31.

———, "Characteristics of the Peripheral Circulatory System," Final Report, Bioengineering Laboratories, U.S. Air Force Academy, 1969.

5 Assisted Circulation

There are many methods of mechanical assistance to aid the failing heart that have been extensively investigated (Cooper and Clark 1968; Goldfarb 1969; Kolff et al. 1969). All the methods attempt to achieve certain hemodynamic objectives. These include decreasing the work of the failing myocardium by reducing the load on the left ventricle, increasing blood flow through the coronary circulation and consequently increasing the oxygen supply to the hypoxic tissue, and increasing cardiac output and thus increasing the blood supply to the peripheral organs (Jaron et al. 1970).

Among the methods of assistance currently under extensive clinical investigation are those using an assist device in series with the left ventricle. A typical temporary device of this type is the so-called balloon pump shown in Figure 5–1 (Moulopolos, Topaz, and Kolff 1962; Kantrowitz et al. 1968). A similar permanent prosthetic unit being investigated is the dynamic aortic patch shown in Figure 5–2 (Kantrowitz et al. 1972). Assist devices of this type periodically produce pressure perturbations in the aorta. Normally the units are driven so that the pressure is elevated during ventricular diastole and lowered prior to ventricular ejection. The effect of the pressure perturbations is to increase the perfusion of the coronary arteries, to increase cardiac output, and to reduce the ejection pressure of the left ventricle. Typical pneumatic driving units for bedside and portable use are shown in Figures 5–3 and 5–4. In addition to pneumatic devices, recent experiments with implantable piezoelectric units show much promise (Williams et al. 1975). Besides in-series diastolic augmentation devices, pumps paralleling the left ventricle have been successfully employed (Liotta et al. 1962).

Such mechanical circulatory assistance appears promising in the management of both chronic and acute forms of medically intractable, progressive left ventricular failure (Kantrowitz et al. 1972). As this application expands, it is becoming apparent that the appropriate automatic control of such devices is of major importance in their proper performance. In order to design apparatus for optimal control functioning, it is necessary to have suitable analytical models which interrelate the device with the heart and circulatory system (Welkowitz et al. 1972). As the applications of mechanical circulatory assistance increase in number and the technology advances, much thought has been given to proper control and optimal adjustment of assist devices. Some effort has already gone into computer control of

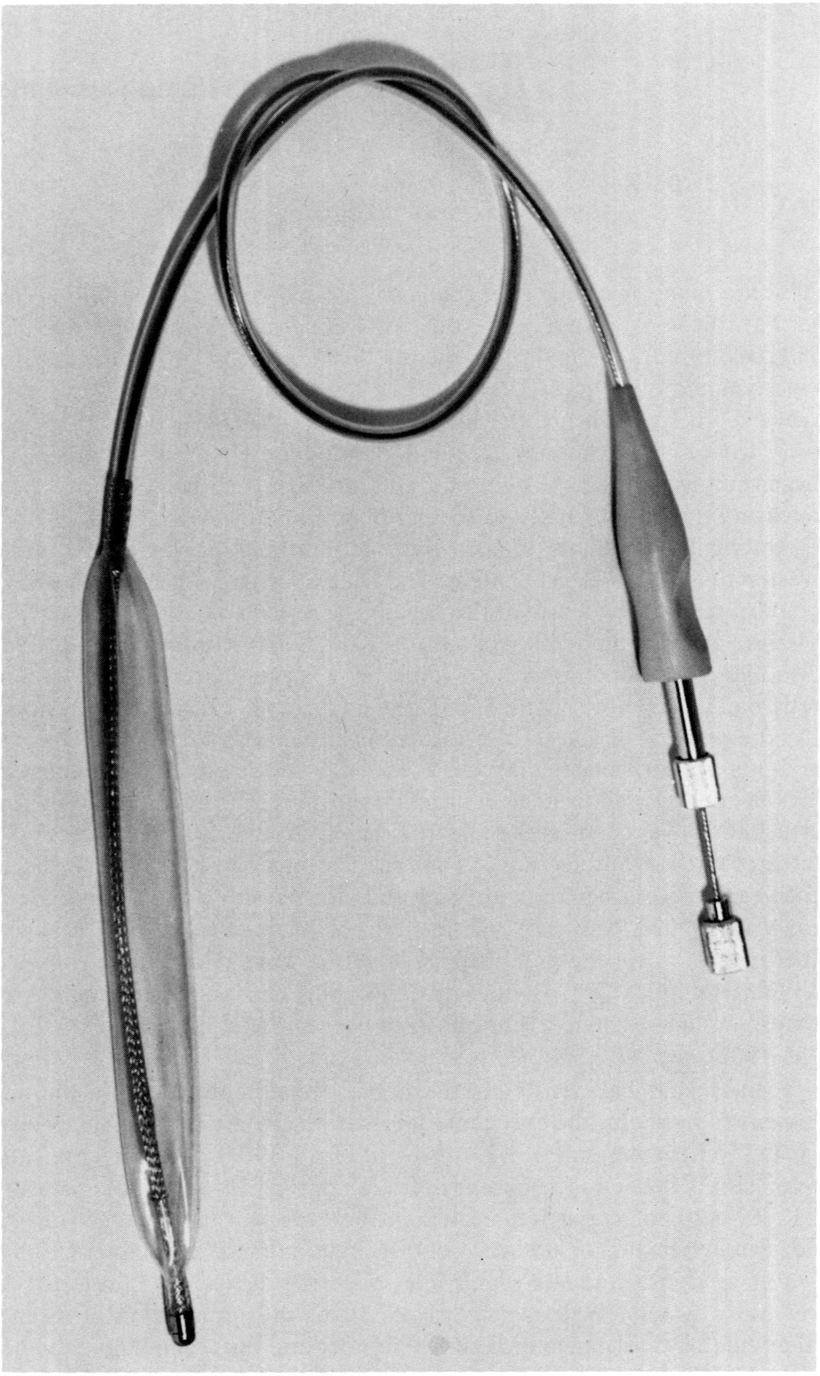

Figure 5–1 Intra-aortic Balloon Pump.

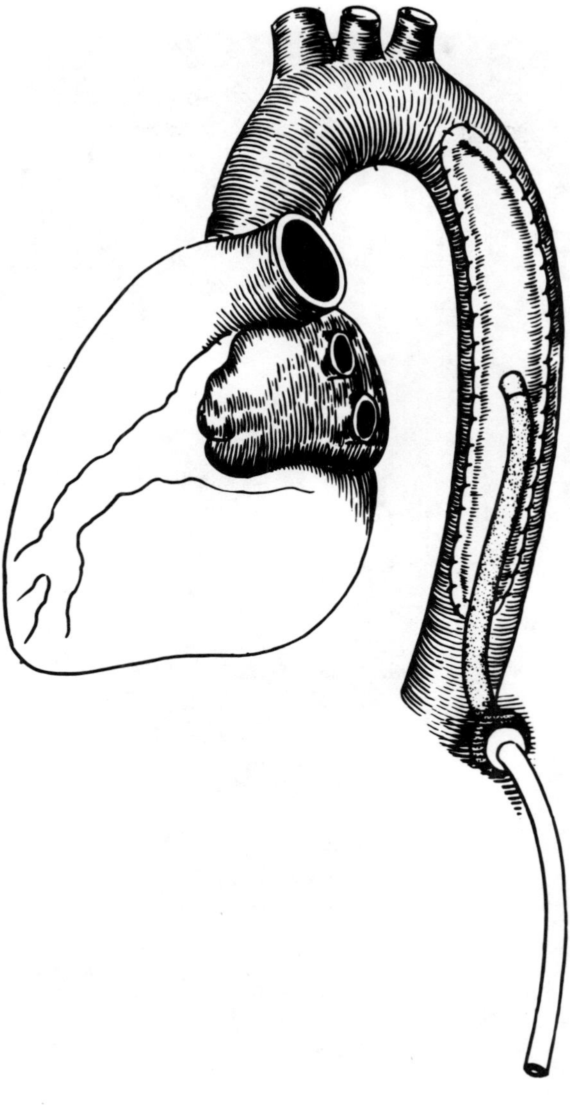

Figure 5–2a Sketch of Inserted Dynamic Aortic Patch

balloon pump operation (Clark 1973; Moskowitz et al. 1976). At the present time, however, most control adjustment is manual and subjective. For example, the controls for the intra-aortic balloon pump are set so that the balloon is inflated at the beginning of the diastolic phase of the heart cycle

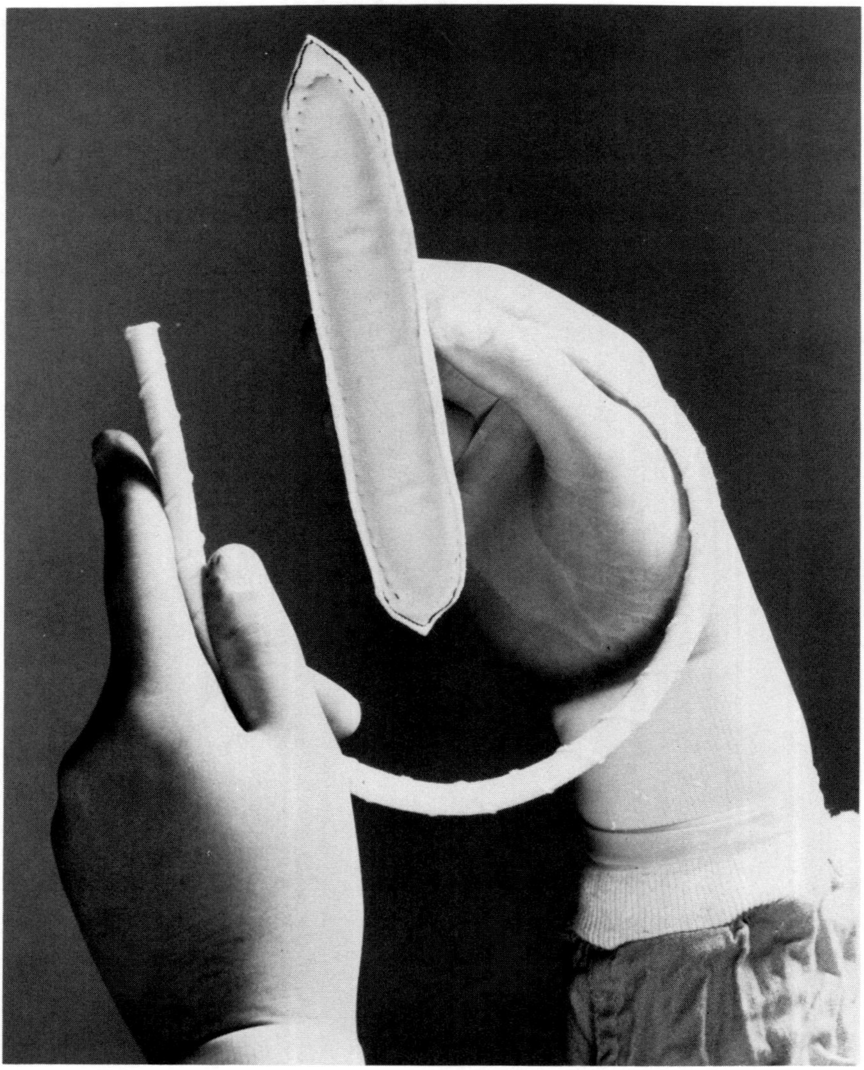

Figure 5–2b Photograph of Dynamic Aortic Patch

and deflated at the end of diastole. This adjustment is made while the central aortic pressure is observed; and, particularly in cases of severe cardiac disease, the appropriate inflation and deflation times are difficult to ascertain. In addition, as the patient recovers, the required adjustments change.

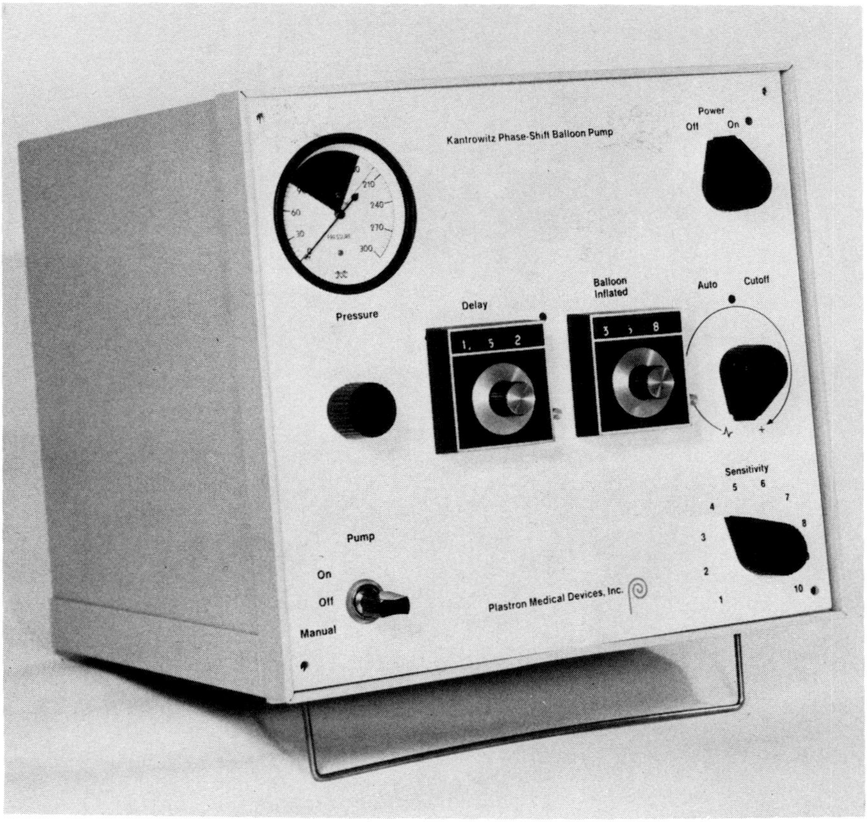

Figure 5–3 Bedside Electropneumatic Driving Unit.

These observations lead to the recognition of the need for more objective criteria for the control and operation of mechanical circulatory assist devices, and in particular for in-series units such as the intra-aortic balloon pump. Algorithms are needed for the selection of suitable patients, for optimal pumping control, and for decisions on termination of pumping. Analytical models of the assisted circulatory system can help in the formulation of these algorithms.

5.1 A Model for Assisted Systemic Circulation

An analytical model which can be used to describe the circulatory assistance procedure has been presented by Welkowitz et al. (1972). The

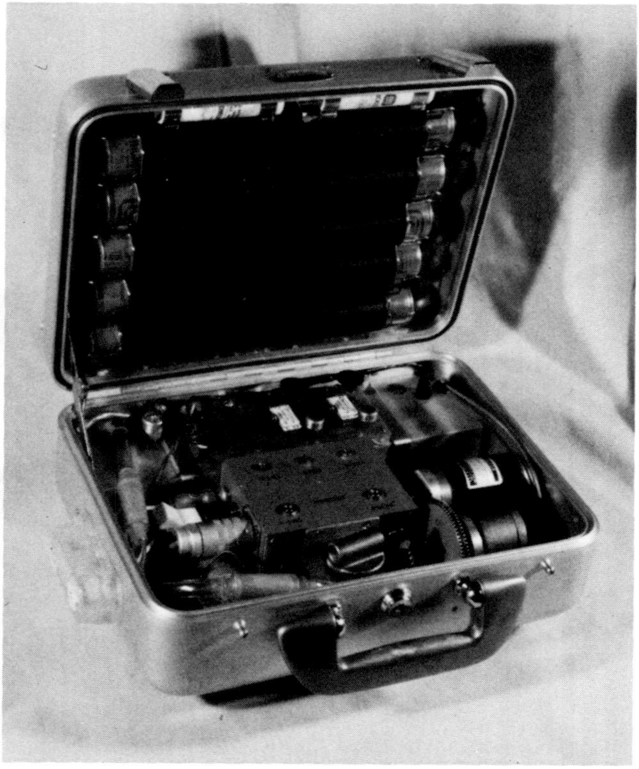

Figure 5–4 Carrying Case Configuration of Motor-compressor Driving Unit.

analytical system consists of submodels of the left ventricle, the aortic valve, the aorta, the peripheral circulatory system, and an in-series assist device located in a region along the aorta. The models for the individual parts of the system have been described in Chapters 2, 3, and 4. The left ventricle is represented by an equivalent pressure source in series with a complex source impedance. The aorta is modeled as a hybrid network consisting of tapered resistive-capacitive distributed sections and a lumped inertance. The peripheral vascular system is considered as a reflectionless termination of the tapered aorta. In accordance with the work of Shastri (1969), the aortic valve, which is a time-varying impedance, is represented by a complex impedance in the frequency domain. Following the suggestion of Shapiro et al. (1969), the in-series device is modeled as a point flow source located at any desired point along the aorta. The use of a point flow

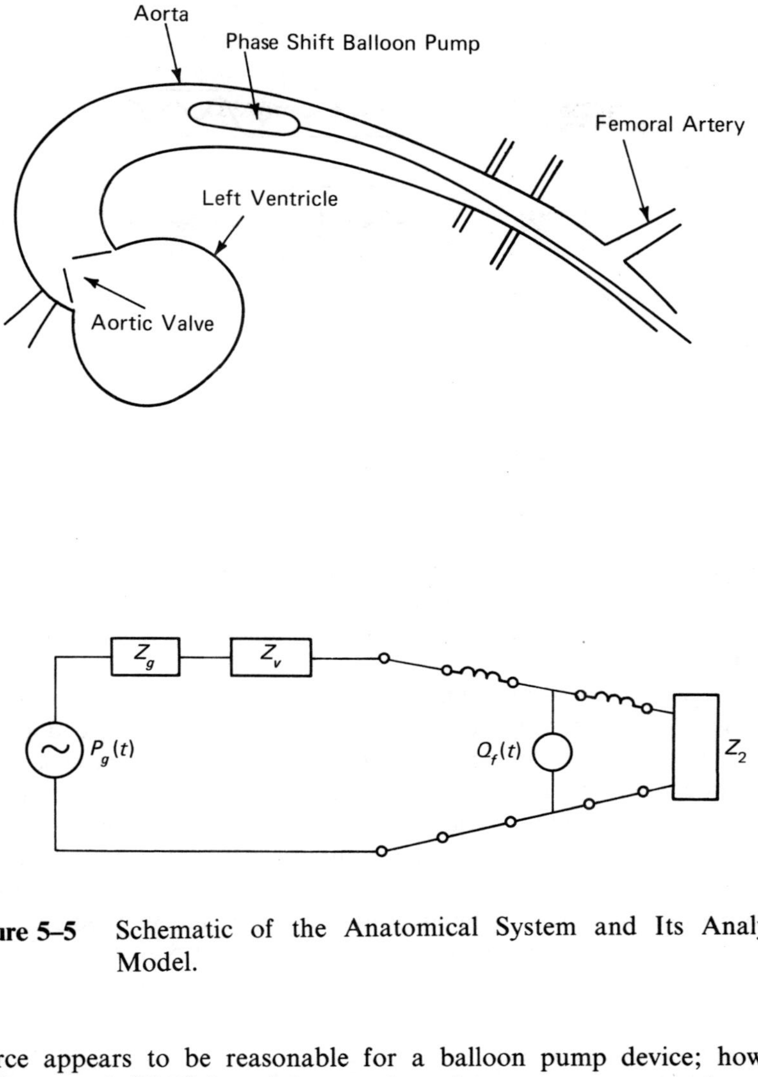

Figure 5–5 Schematic of the Anatomical System and Its Analytical Model.

source appears to be reasonable for a balloon pump device; however, Williams et al. (1975) found the use of a point pressure source to be a more suitable representation of a pressure-generating unit such as a piezoelectric assist device. A schematic of the vascular system and its model equivalent is shown in Figure 5–5. As suggested, the flow source $Q_f(t)$ can be replaced by a pressure source $P_f(t)$ when appropriate.

The initial analysis and the development of performance criteria using the system of Figure 5–5 are carried out at the heart fundamental frequency (or heart rate). However, since the model chosen is assumed to be linear, similar calculations can be carried out for the average terms and higher

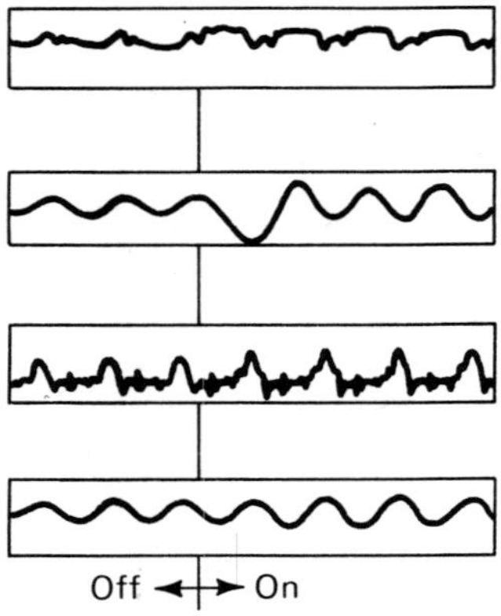

Figure 5–6 Fundamental Components of Pressure and Flow Waves—Pumping and Nonpumping.

harmonics. Then desired time-domain waveforms can be calculated by superposition. In the dynamic optimization problem considered later in this chapter, the average terms as well as the fundamental frequency terms are utilized.

In order to establish the validity of some of the results obtained from the model of Figure 5–5, experiments were performed on mongrel dogs with inserted intra-aortic balloon pumps. Data were taken of ventricular pressure, aortic flow and pressure, and aortic geometry. These data permit calculations of the model parameters. In addition, electronic filters were used with the aortic flow and aortic pressure signals to measure directly the amplitude and phase of the fundamental waves. These waveforms are the output signals that were compared to the initial model predictions. A typical recording of measured data is shown in Figure 5–6.

5.1.1 Analysis of the Model

The left ventricle equivalent source model is described in Chapter 2, and the values of the phasors P_g and Z_g can be obtained from Eqs. (2–5) and (2–6). The aorta network model is described in Chapter 3, and the transmission properties can be obtained from Eqs. (3–39) through (3–48). The terminating impedance for no reflection is given in Eq. (3–46).

Since the system is approximately described by the linear network of Figure 5–5, the operating characteristics at the fundamental frequency can be determined by considering the network as a two-pump system and using the principle of superposition. The superposition model is shown in Figure 5–7. For the case of the ventricle operating alone, Figure 5–7*a* applies. For the case of the auxiliary pump operating alone, Figure 5–7*b* applies. Let us employ the following notation for the phasor quantities:

Z_{11} = aortic input impedance without pumping
P_{11} = aortic root pressure without pumping
Q_{11} = aortic root flow without pumping
Q_f = ideal flow-source flow
P_f = pressure at the ideal source operating alone
P_{12} = aortic root pressure with pump source operating alone; no heart source
Q_{12} = aortic flow with pump source operating alone; no heart source
P_1 = total aortic root pressure
Q_1 = total aortic root flow
$\begin{vmatrix} A_T & B_T \\ C_T & D_T \end{vmatrix}$ = transmission matrix of the section of aorta to the pump source

Then, referring to Figure 5–7*a*, we have

$$P_{11} = \frac{P_g Z_{11}}{Z_{11} + Z_g + Z_v} \tag{5–1}$$

$$Q_{11} = \frac{P_g}{Z_{11} + Z_g + Z_v} \tag{5–2}$$

Referring to Figure 5–7*b*, we get

$$P_{12} = A_T P_f + B_T Q_f \tag{5–3}$$

$$Q_{12} = C_T P_f + D_T Q_f \tag{5–4}$$

$$P_{12} = Q_{12}(Z_g + Z_v) \tag{5–5}$$

Combining these three equations to eliminate P_f yields

$$P_{12} = \left\{-\frac{A_T[B_T + D_T(Z_g + Z_v)]}{A_T + C_T(Z_g + Z_v)} + B_T\right\}Q_f \tag{5–6}$$

$$Q_{12} = \frac{1}{Z_g + Z_v}\left\{\frac{A_T[B_T + D_T(Z_g + Z_v)]}{A_T + C_T(Z_g + Z_v)} - B_T\right\}Q_f \tag{5–7}$$

Using the principle of superposition gives

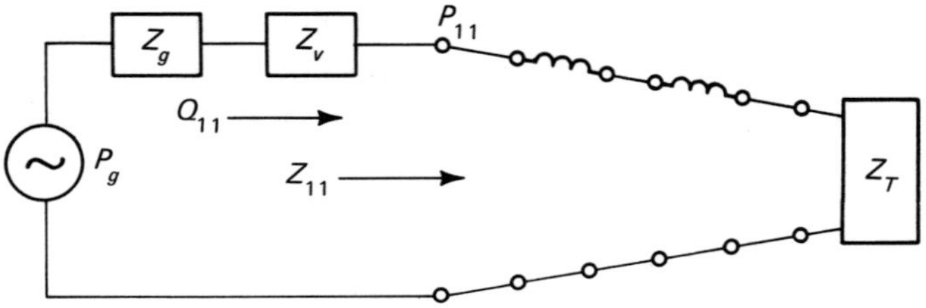

(a)

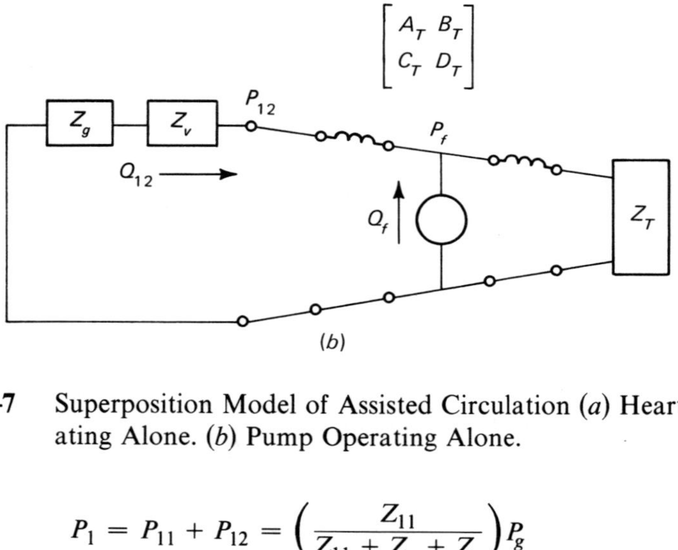

(b)

Figure 5–7 Superposition Model of Assisted Circulation (*a*) Heart Operating Alone. (*b*) Pump Operating Alone.

$$P_1 = P_{11} + P_{12} = \left(\frac{Z_{11}}{Z_{11} + Z_g + Z_v}\right) P_g - \left\{\frac{A_T[B_T + D_T(Z_g + Z_v)]}{A_T + C_T(Z_g + Z_v)} - B_T\right\} Q_f \tag{5–8}$$

$$Q_1 = Q_{11} + Q_{12} = \frac{1}{Z_{11} + Z_g + Z_v} P_g + \frac{1}{Z_g + Z_v}\left\{\frac{A_T[B_T + D_T(Z_g + Z_v)]}{A_T + C_T(Z_g + Z_v)} - B_T\right\} Q_f \tag{5–9}$$

Equations (5–8) and (5–9) relate total aortic pressure P_1 and total aortic flow Q_1 to the left ventricular source pressure P_g and to the flow from the ideal flow source Q_f.

5.1.2 *Initial Applications of This Model*

Experimental work on dogs (Jaron et al. 1970) suggests that one criterion for optimal physiological pumping is that the fundamental component of aortic pressure and the fundamental component of aortic flow be 180° out of phase with each other during pumping. The dependence of some of the system characteristics on this phase angle can be calculated readily from the equations developed. Thus one can calculate (1) equivalent source power (for the fundamental components)

$$W_g = |P_g||Q_1|\cos\theta_{g1} \tag{5–10}$$

where θ_{g1} is the phase angle between P_g and Q_1, and (2) aortic power (for the fundamental components)

$$W_a = |P_1||Q_1|\cos\theta_{11} \tag{5–11}$$

where θ_{11} is the phase angle between P_1 and Q_1.

These parameters can be plotted against the aortic impedance fundamental component phase angle θ_{11}. An examination of the quantities in these equations indicates that some specific source parameter and aorta parameter values must be utilized in the theoretical calculations. Typical values from an experiment on an anesthetized dog are shown in Table 5–1. The resultant theoretical curves of source power and aortic power calculated from Eqs. (5–10) and (5–11) are shown in Figures 5–8 and 5–9.

Various experiments were performed to investigate these theoretical relationships. A typical experimental curve of aortic power reduction versus

Table 5–1
Heart and Aorta Parameters, Experiment 108

Heart Parameters—Fundamental Components	
$P_g = 31 \times 10^3 \text{N/m}^2$	
$\theta_{pg} = 2.80$ rad	
$Z_g = 2.0 \times 10^8$ Ns/m^5	
$\theta_{zg} = -3.13$ rad	
Aorta Parameters—Measured and Calculated	
Length to pump	0.13 m
Length from pump to bifurcation	0.34 m
Taper coefficient	2.5m^{-1}
Input area	$3.1 \times 10^{-4}\text{m}^2$
Aortic root hoop elasticity	$9.3 \times 10^4\text{N/m}^2$
Heart Rate	
150 bpm	

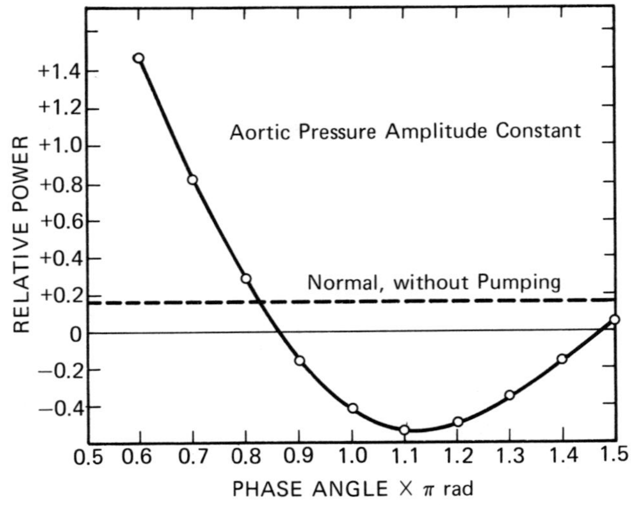

Figure 5–8 Calculated Change in Pulsatile Fundamental Component of Source Work versus Aortic Impedance Phase Angle (Constant Pressure).

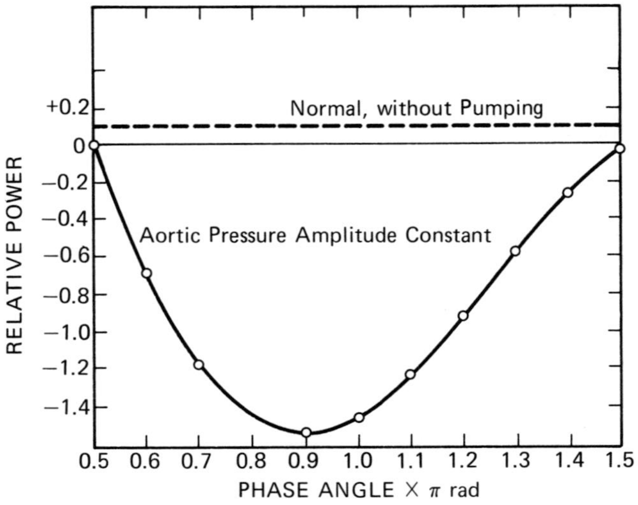

Figure 5–9 Calculated Change in Pulsatile Fundamental Component of Aortic Work versus Aortic Impedance Phase Angle (Constant Pressure).

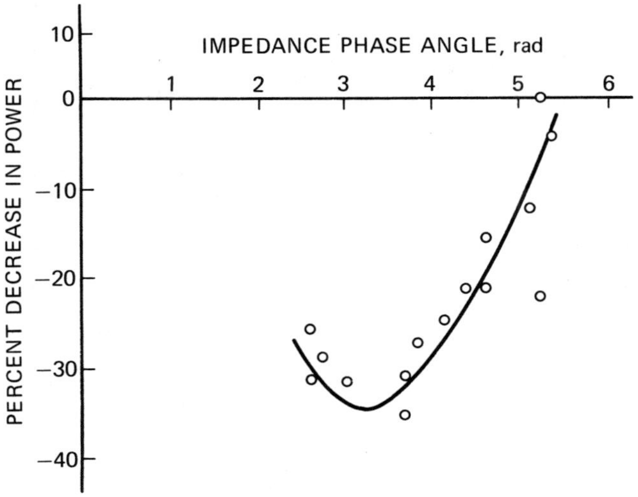

Figure 5–10 Experimental Reduction of Pulsatile Fundamental Component of Aortic Work versus Aortic Impedance Phase Angle.

aortic impedance phase angle from one of these experiments (Jaron et al. 1970) is shown in Figure 5–10. A comparison of Figures 5–9 and 5–10 shows that both the experimental and the theoretical minima occur at approximately the same phase angle, θ_{11}. This agreement of both theory and experiment tends to support strongly the phase angle criterion (approximately 180° phase shift) as an operating condition for optimal pumping.

Further verification experiments were carried out on the dog with the anatomical data shown in Table 5–1. Figure 5–11 is a plot of the amplitude of the fundamental component of aortic flow versus the amplitude of the fundamental component of aortic pressure for a fixed phase angle between them ($\theta_{11} = 0.78\pi$ rad). Calculations from the model using the data of Table 5–1 are plotted on the same figure. Figure 5–12 is a plot of measured aortic power versus the amplitude of the fundamental component of aortic pressure for a constant fundamental frequency impedance phase angle ($\theta_{11} = 0.78\pi$ rad). Again calculations from the model are plotted on the same figure. The good agreement observed between measurement and calculation supports the applicability of the model of Figure 5–5 to the analysis of assisted circulation.

Using a similar model with a point pressure source substituted for the flow source, Williams (1975) investigated the effects of device position along the aorta on the efficacy of mechanical circulatory assistance. He calculated

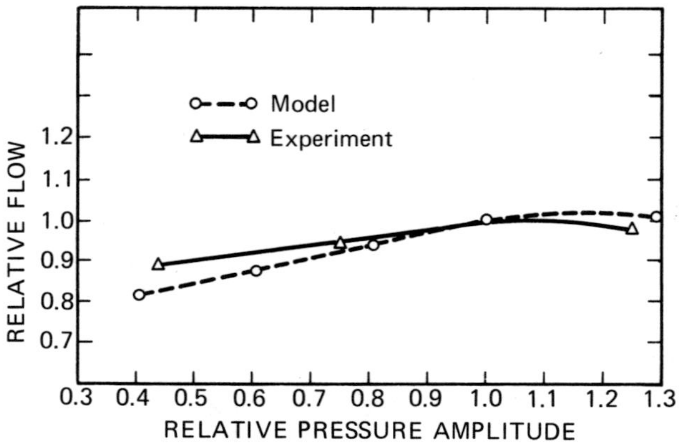

Figure 5–11 Relative Aortic Flow versus Pressure Amplitude; Comparison of Model and Experiment.

required device pressure to produce the same fundamental component of aortic root pressure as the device was moved distally from the heart. The results, as shown in Figure 5–13, suggest that the device pressure must be increased about 40 percent if it is moved from a location near the aortic root to the lower abdominal aorta. Thus, variations in device location must be accompanied by changes in device driving power.

5.2 Dynamic Optimization

Thus far the model analyzed has been used to support the applicability of the 180° phase shift operating criterion. In addition, it has been used to suggest the variation in device power requirement as a function of location along the aorta and to support the measured functional variation of aortic power reduction and aortic flow with variations in device-driving amplitude. These latter two observations were primarily verifications to increase the acceptability of the model. With confidence in the model, it can be used to explore both the possibility of dynamic optimization of the control adjustments while pumping is in progress and the determination of criteria for terminating pumping.

Before the optimization procedure is explored in detail, it is necessary to extend the model described by Figure 5–5 and Eqs. (5–1) through (5–9) to include the average (or mean) terms. For these average terms the equations analogous to Eqs. (5–8) and (5–9) are

$$P'_1 = \frac{R_{ai} + R_{aT}}{(R_s + R_v + R_{ai} + R_{aT})} P_s + \frac{(R_s + R_v)(R_x + R_{aT})}{(R_s + R_v + R_{ai} + R_{aT})} Q'_f \qquad (5\text{–}12)$$

$$Q'_1 = \frac{R_{ai} + R_{aT}}{(R_s + R_v + R_{ai} + R_{aT})} P_s - \frac{(R_{aT} + R_x)}{(R_s + R_v + R_{ai} + R_{aT})} Q'_f \qquad (5\text{–}13)$$

where P'_1 = average aortic root pressure during assisted circulation
Q'_1 = average aortic root flow during assisted circulation
P_s = average value of the equivalent left ventricle pressure source
R_s = equivalent left ventricle internal resistance
R_v = equivalent valve resistance
R_{ai} = series input resistance of the aorta
R_{aT} = series resistance of the aorta termination
R_x = equivalent series aortic resistance for the section of the aorta between the assist device and the femoral bifurcation
Q'_f = average assist device flow

The two different loading conditions on the heart, obtained by the action of the assist device, are used to calculate the values of the lumped parameters P_s and R_s as well as the fundamental frequency phasors of the

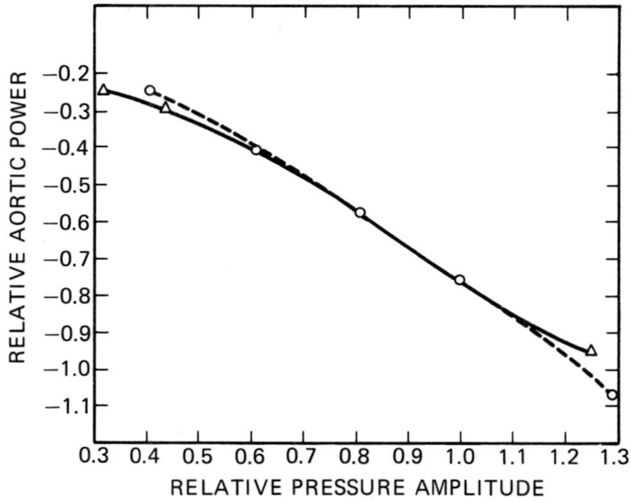

Figure 5–12 Relative Aortic Work versus Pressure Amplitude; Comparison of Model and Experiment.

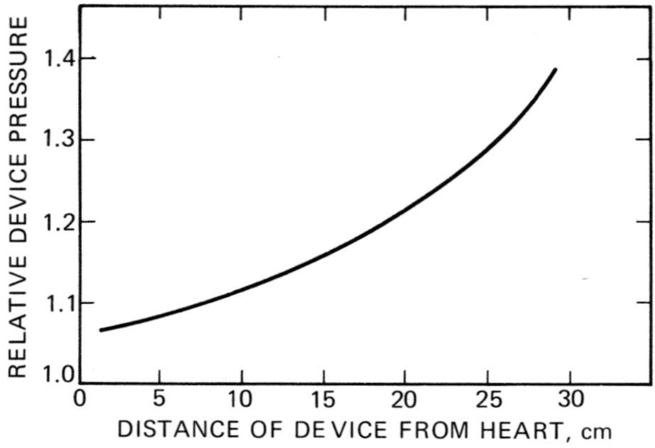

Figure 5–13 Effect of Location of Assist Device along the Aorta on Required Device Pressure.

source parameters P_g and Z_g. Min (1972) also used these fundamental phasors to calculate a spatially averaged maximum isovolumic wall stress for the left ventricle. The value of this stress component in terms of the magnitudes of the source fundamental frequency phasors is given by

$$\sigma_{av} = K_p \frac{P_{gm}}{\sqrt{Z_{gm}}} \tag{5–14}$$

where K_p is a constant. σ_{av} represents a measure of the capability of the left ventricle muscle wall to develop pressure or to produce work.

5.2.1 Pumping Performance Criteria

The purpose of the optimization procedures that are described in this section is to minimize a performance index which is defined by objective criteria (Min et al. 1975): This performance index is composed of two terms: (1) the time integral of left ventricular power divided by the calculated maximum isovolumic stress as defined by Eq. (5–14) and (2) a weighted terminal constraint index, which is defined as the weighted difference between the desired hemodynamic conditions and the actual hemodynamic conditions at the end of mechanical assistance. Based upon the discussions in the previous section, a boundary condition constraint was added to the performance criteria forcing the phase angle of the aorta input impedance at the fundamental frequency to be held at π rad.

Table 5–2
Effect of Intra-aortic Balloon Pumping on the "Normalized" Heart Work of a Failing Heart

Experiment Number	*Ratio of Left Ventricle Hemodynamic Power to Calculated Maximum Isovolumic Stress*		(2)/(1)
	After Ligation (1)	*After Therapeutic Pumping* (2)	
502	0.67	0.56	84%
503	0.60	0.48	80%
504	1.30	1.00	77%
505	0.50	0.24	48%
506	0.89	0.56	63%

In the initial investigations of optimized pumping, the minimization of total left ventricular work over the pumping period was chosen as an important physiological criterion. Further theoretical and experimental studies of mechanical assistance demonstrated that this modality changes the length-tension-velocity relationship of heart muscle (Min 1972). Therefore the ratio of left ventricular power to calculated isovolumic stress was chosen instead as the variable of interest. As indicated in Table 5–2, this ratio is consistently reduced in pumping experiments designed to aid the left ventricle.

The choice of the terminal constraint index as a performance criterion was based upon one of the major objectives of mechanical assistance, namely, to return the hemodynamic parameters measured in the aorta,such as pressure and flow, close to the "normal" values. This is particularly an objective for patients in cardiogenic shock. Thus, the deviations of the average and the fundamental pulsatile values of aortic pressure and flow from "normal" values have been chosen as one component of the performance index.

The *total performance index* is defined as the sum of the "normalized" left ventricular work and the weighted square of the deviations of the aorta hemodynamic parameters.

5.2.2 Optimization Procedure

The optimization procedure finds an optimal, multistage control function such that the hemodynamic conditions of the circulatory system approach the desired conditions with minimum left ventricular energy expenditure. A state-variable equation technique is utilized in the analysis. The duration of mechanical assistance is divided into n discrete stages (or periods). The optimization procedure consists of defining the system states at each of

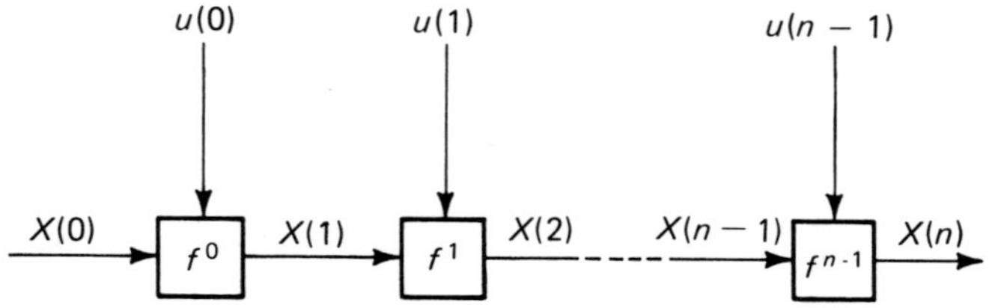

Figure 5–14 Multistage Dynamic System.

these stages and minimizing the performance index during the transition from stage to stage.

A diagram of the multistage dynamic system is shown in Figure 5–14. The aortic pressure and flow conditions are chosen as state variables $X(k)$. The assist device flow conditions are chosen as the control variables $u(k)$. The state and control variables are defined within this framework as follows:

$X(1, k) =$ k-stage magnitude of the fundamental component of aortic pressure in the ascending aorta
$X(2, k) =$ k-stage phase angle of the fundamental component of the aortic pressure
$X(3, k) =$ k-stage magnitude of the fundamental component of aortic flow in the ascending aorta
$X(4, k) =$ k-stage average aortic pressure
$X(5, k) =$ k stage average aortic flow
$u(1, k) =$ k-stage magnitude of the fundamental component of assist device input flow
$u(2, k) =$ k-stage phase angle of the fundamental component of assist device input flow
$u(3, k) =$ k-stage average assist device input flow

At each stage the control vector u determines the transition of the state variables from $X(k)$ to $X(k + 1)$. The system is initially in a known state of failure $X(0)$, a five-dimensional state vector. The initial setting of the flow assist device defines a three-dimensional control vector $u(0)$ which determines the transition to a state described as $X(1)$ through the functional relationship f^0 as follows:

$$X(1) = f^0[X(0), u(0)] \tag{5–15}$$

In general, the $(k + 1)$-stage state variables are derived from the k-stage state variables through the relationship

$$X(k+1) = f^k[X(k), u(k)] \tag{5–16}$$

For optimal operation, the pump control variables $u(0)$, $u(1)$, ..., $u(n-1)$ should be adjusted to minimize the normalized heart work in such a manner that state variables $X(k)$ approach normal aortic hemodynamic conditions in n stages.

The functional relationships f^k are defined from the model of Figures 5–5 and 5–6 and Eqs. (5–8), (5–9), (5–12), and (5–13). When expressed as difference equations, these become

$$\begin{aligned} X(1,k+1) = \{&X^2(1,k) + B_{Zm}{}^2(k)u^2(1,k) \\ &- 2X(1,k)B_{Zm}(k)u(1,k) \\ &\cdot \cos[X(2,k) - \theta_{Zb}(k) - u(2,k)]\}^{1/2} \end{aligned} \tag{5–17}$$

$$X(2,k+1) = \tan^{-1}\left\{\frac{X(1,k)\sin[X(2,k)] - B_{Zm}(k)u(1,k)\sin[\theta_{Zb}(k) + u(2,k)]}{X(1,k)\cos[X(2,k)] - B_{Zm}(k)u(1,k)\cos[\theta_{Zb}(k) + u(2,k)]}\right\} \tag{5–18}$$

$$\begin{aligned} X(3,k+1) = \{&X^2(3,k) + D_{Zm}{}^2(k)u^2(1,k) \\ &- 2D_{Zm}(k)X(3,k)u(1,k) \\ &\cdot \cos[X(2,k) - \theta_{Zd}(k) - u(2,k)]\}^{1/2} \end{aligned} \tag{5–19}$$

$$X(4,k+1) = X(4,k) + \frac{[R_{aT}(k) + R_x(k)][R_s(k) + R_v(k)]}{P_s(k)} X(5,k)u(3,k) \tag{5–20}$$

$$X(5,k+1) = X(5,k) - \frac{R_{aT}(k) + R_x(k)}{[R_{ai}(k) + R_{aT}(k)]P_s(k)} X(4,k)u(3,k) \tag{5–21}$$

In Eqs. (5–17) to (5–21), four complex variables A_Z, B_Z, C_Z, and D_Z are defined as follows:

$$A_Z = A_{Zm}e^{j\theta_{Za}} = \frac{Z_{11}}{Z_{11} + Z_g + Z_v} \tag{5–22}$$

$$B_Z = B_{Zm}e^{j\theta_{Zb}} = \frac{A_T[B_T + D_T(Z_g + Z_v)]}{A_T C_T(Z_g + Z_v)} - B_T \tag{5–23}$$

$$C_Z = C_{Zm}e^{j\theta_{Zc}} = \frac{1}{Z_g + Z_v + Z_{11}} \tag{5–24}$$

$$D_Z = D_{Zm} e^{j\theta_{Zd}} = \frac{1}{Z_g + Z_v} B_T \tag{5–25}$$

The state-variable equations (5–17) through (5–21) incorporate the boundary condition which forces the phase angle of the input impedance of the aorta at the fundamental frequency to be π rad.

In the state-variable notation the components of the performance index can be expressed as follows. (1) *Normalized left ventricular work*:

$$J_1 = \sum_{k=1}^{n-1} \frac{1}{P_{gm}^2(k)/Z_{gm}(k)} \left\{ \frac{X(1,k)}{A_{Zm}(k)} \left[X(3,k)\cos\theta_{Zc}(k) \right.\right.$$
$$+ D_{Zm}(k)u(1,k)\cos[\theta_g(k) - \theta_{Zd}(k) - u(2,k)] + [P_s(k)X(5,k)$$
$$\left.\left. - \frac{R_{aT}(k) + R_x(k)}{R_{ai}(k) + R_{aT}(k)} X(4,k)u(3,k) \right] \right\}^2 \tag{5–26}$$

(2) *terminal constraint*:

$$J_2 = w1[XF1 - X(1,n)]^2 + w2[XF2 - X(2,n)]^2 + w3[XF3 - X(3,n)]^2$$
$$+ w4[XF4 - X(4,n)]^2 + w5[XF5 - X(5,n)]^2 \tag{5–27}$$

where P_{gm} = magnitude of P_g
Z_{gm} = magnitude of Z_g
XFi = desired aortic hemodynamic condition (condition prior to heart failure); $i = 1, 2, \ldots, 5$
wi = weighting constant; $i = 1, 2, \ldots, 5$

The total performance index is then

$$J = J_1 + J_2 \tag{5–28}$$

The choice of weighting constants was done primarily by numerical experimentation.

An iterative-search algorithm has been developed to minimize the performance index of Eq. (5–28) at each state transition. Using the state-variable equations, Fletcher and Reeve's (1964) conjugate gradient search method is employed to find the function minima. A quadratic interpolation technique (Fox 1971) is used to determine the step size. The gradients used in the search method can be evaluated by employing Bryson and Ho's development (1971) of the dynamic multiage optimal control problem. The adjoint system equation can then be evaluated using the method of Lagrange multipliers (Lee, Adams, and Gaines 1971). Equation (5–28) can be expressed in the following functional form by using Eqs. (5–26) and (5–27):

$$J = \phi[X(N)] + \sum_{k=0}^{N-1} L^k[X(k), u(k)] \tag{5–29}$$

where ϕ and L^k are functions given by Eqs. (5–26) and (5–27). By combining Eq. (5–29) and Eq. (5–16), the gradient of a Hamiltonian function and the Lagrange multiplier can be defined as

$$\frac{\partial H^k}{\partial u(k)} = \frac{\partial L^k}{\partial u(k)} + \lambda^{T_m}(k+1)\frac{\partial f^k}{\partial u(k)} \tag{5–30}$$

$$\lambda(k) = \left[\frac{\partial f^k}{\partial X(k)}\right]^{T_m} \lambda(k+1) + \left[\frac{\partial L^k}{\partial X(k)}\right]^{T_m} \tag{5–31}$$

$$\lambda(N) = \left[\frac{\partial \phi}{\partial X(N)}\right]^{T_m} \tag{5–32}$$

where T_m = the transpose—T_m in $[\partial f^k/\partial X(k)]^{T_m}$ denotes the transpose of a matrix
H^k = a Hamiltonian function
$\lambda(k)$ = the Lagrange multiplier, $k = 0, 1, 2, \ldots, n-1$
$X(0)$ = the initial hemodynamic condition in the aorta after ventricular failure

Using Eqs. (5–30) through (5–32), the computer algorithm diagramed in Figure 5–15 was developed to find the optimal pump control function and the subsequent time-domain functions for the aortic hemodynamic conditions. The results obtainable for a single-stage transition using the algorithm of Figure 5–15 are exemplified by Figure 5–16 in which the fundamental components of aortic root flow and assist device flow are plotted for the transition from the j to the $(j+1)$ stage.

5.2.3 Experimental Verification

Real-time optimization using the procedure developed has not been attempted yet. However, off-line computations have been carried out and compared with measurements on dogs with experimentally induced myocardial infarctions which were permitted to go into cardiogenic shock and then were treated therapeutically by means of intra-aortic balloon pumping. The driving system adjustments in these experiments were carried out by experienced personnel utilizing subjective examinations of the central aortic pressure waveforms. In these experiments the aortic pressure and flow before coronary artery ligation were defined as the desired hemodynamic

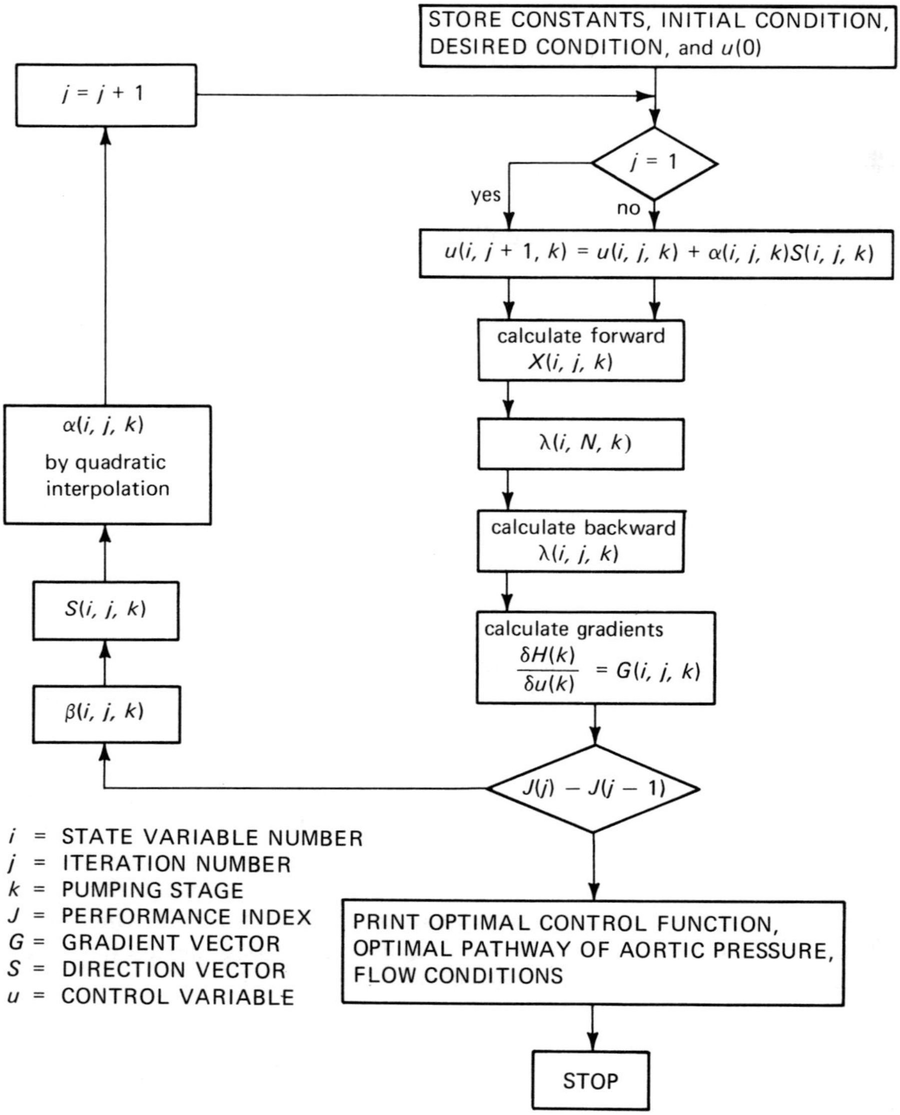

Figure 5–15 Flow Diagram for Calculation of Optimal Pump Control Function.

conditions in the terminal constraint portion of the performance index. The pressure and flow conditions after left ventricular failure had been induced, and before the start of mechanical assistance, were used as the initial

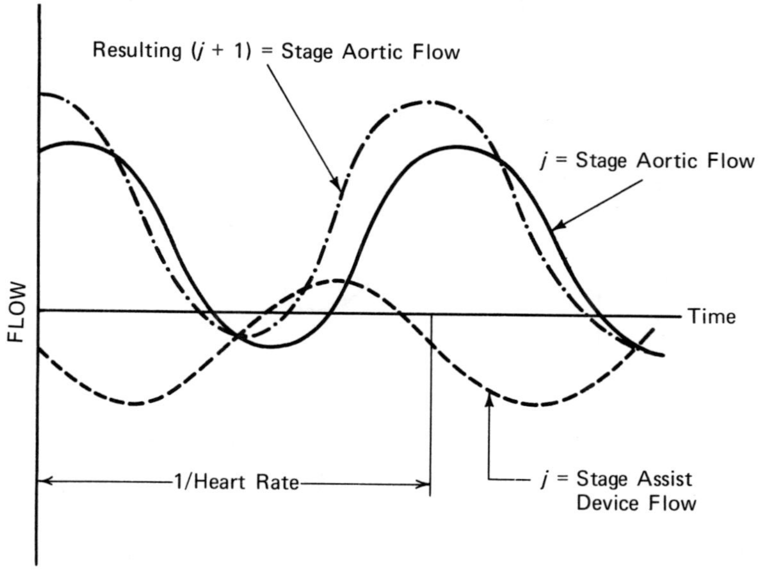

Figure 5–16 Fundamental Components of Aortic Root Flow and Calculated Optimal Assist Device Flow.

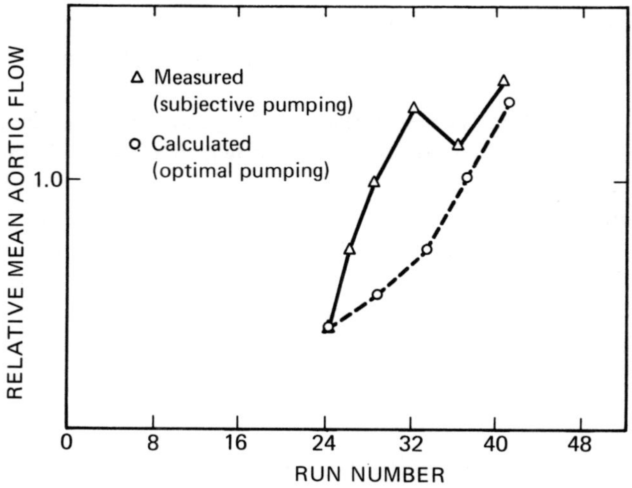

Note: There is an equal time between runs of approximately 3 minutes. This applies to figures 5-18 and 5-21 through 5-25.

Figure 5–17 Experimental and Calculated Values of Mean Aortic Flow as a Function of Time, Experiment 502.

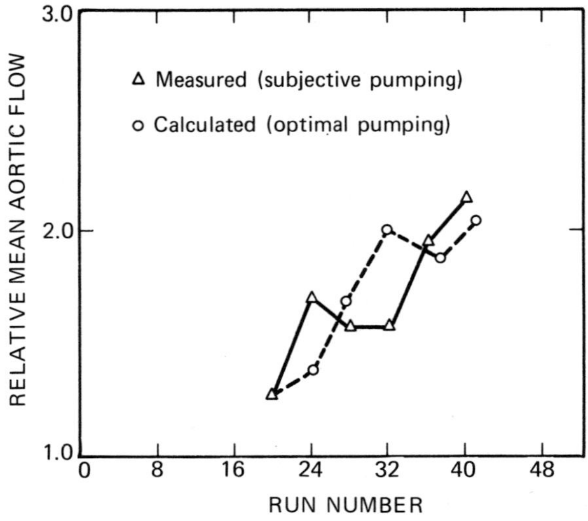

Figure 5–18 Experimental and Calculated Values of Mean Aortic Flow as a Function of Time, Experiment 504.

conditions in the optimization calculations. "Normalized" heart work was used as the other portion of the performance index. Typical time functions of mean aortic flow from two of these experiments are shown in Figures 5–17 and 5–18. In these figures, the subjective experimental pumping hemodynamic values are compared with values calculated using the optimization algorithm.

A more comprehensive comparison of the optimization calculations and the results from these two experiments is shown in Tables 5–3 and 5–4. The weighting constants used in these calculations were arrived at by a combination of numerical analysis and numerical experimentation. Further experimentation is needed to establish definitive weighting constants. In these tables both components of the final value of the performance index are shown. The optimization algorithm yielded lower values for each segment, suggesting that better pump control would improve the physiological effectiveness of mechanical assistance.

5.2.4 *Applications to Computer Control of Pumping*

The purpose of the work presented in Section 5.2.3 was to develop analytical techniques which would permit more objective control of assist device driving systems as an improvement over the present subjective

Table 5–3

A Comparison of Subjectively Adjusted Experimental Mechanical Assistance and Calculated Optimal Performance Criteria, Experiment 502

Parameters	*State Variable*	*Initial Aortic Condition*	*Desired Aortic Condition (XF)*	*Final Aortic Condition X(n)*		*Terminal Constraints Index* wi$[XF - X(n)]^2$			*Ratio* $\left(\frac{Sub.}{Opt.}\right)$
				Sub.	*Opt.*	*wi*	*Sub.*	*Opt.*	
Aortic pressure, flow condition	P_{1m}	0.18	0.58	0.28	0.67	0.08	72×10^{-4}	6.5×10^{-4}	
	θ_p	−2.80	−2.83	3.03	−1.60	3×10^{-4}	105×10^{-4}	6.0×10^{-4}	
	Q_{1m}	0.80	1.65	1.30	1.12	0.17	0.021	0.485	
	P'	2.72	5.60	3.96	5.49	0.60	1.55	0.006	
	Q'	0.39	1.35	1.41	1.33	1.00	3×10^{-3}	4×10^{-4}	
	sum						1.59	0.49	3.25
Normalized heart work criterion							2.45	1.03	2.38
Total performance index							4.04	1.52	2.65

P_{1m} = fundamental component magnitude of pulsatile aortic pressure (20 mm Hg/unit)
θ_p = fundamental component phase angle of pulsatile aortic pressure (rad)
Q_{1m} = fundamental component magnitude of pulsatile aortic flow (1.5 *l*/min/unit)
P' = mean value of aortic pressure (20 mm Hg/unit)

Q' = mean value of aortic flow (1.5 *l*/min/unit)
Sub. = subjectively controlled experimental pumping
Opt. = calculated optimal pumping
wi = weighting factors

Table 5–4

A Comparison of Subjectively Adjusted Experimental Mechanical Assistance and Calculated Optimal Performance Criteria, Experiment 504

Parameters	*State Variable*	*Initial Aortic Condition*	*Desired Aortic Condition* (XF)	*Final Aortic Condition* $X(n)$		*Terminal Constraint Index* $wi[XF - X(n)]^2$			*Ratio* $\left(\frac{Sub.}{Opt.}\right)$
				Sub.	*Opt.*	*wi*	*Sub.*	*Opt.*	
Aortic pressure, flow condition	P_{1m}	0.98	0.65	0.60	0.76	19.6	0.05	0.19	
	θ_p	2.30	3.04	2.81	2.48	2.3	0.12	0.75	
	Q_{1m}	0.75	1.44	1.61	1.54	13.8	0.4	0.14	
	P'	5.67	5.75	5.27	6.00	1.6	0.37	0.10	
	Q'	0.26	0.91	1.06	1.00	65.0	1.5	0.53	
	sum						2.44	1.71	1.43
Normalized heart work criterion							3.65	2.00	1.83
Total performance index							6.09	3.71	1.65

P_{1m} = fundamental component magnitude of pulsatile aortic pressure (20 mm Hg/unit)
θ_p = fundamental component phase angle of pulsatile aortic pressure (rad)
Q_{1m} = fundamental component magnitude of pulsatile aortic flow (1.5 *l*/min/unit)
P' = mean value of aortic pressure (20 mm Hg/unit)
Q' = mean value of aortic flow (1.5 *l*/min/unit)
Sub. = subjectively controlled experimental pumping
Opt. = calculated optimal pumping
wi = weighting factors

adjustment techniques. The comparisons between experimental therapeutic cardiac mechanical assistance and the optimization calculations suggest that it would be worthwhile to investigate online computer control of pumping in which the computer evaluates the measurements, calculates the optimal control functions as described, and appropriately adjusts the assist device.

The dynamic optimal control technique described has the advantage over other methods that it takes into account the inaccuracies of the physiological simulation and the effects of uncontrolled variables. The calculated optimal state variables are compared against the measured state variables at corresponding time intervals. The measured state variables can be used as new initial conditions for the input of the optimal control program if the difference between predicted and measured state variables is significant.

In this optimal control problem, the performance index specifications need not actually be achieved. They can represent goals that one attempts to reach by means of the control functions (Min et al. 1975). These control functions should improve the performance index with each stage of pumping.

5.3 The Role of Cardiac Control Mechanisms in Assisted Circulation

The physiological effects of assisted circulation can be intuitively explained by considering the in-series assist device as a simple pump in series with the left ventricle. However, clinical studies have demonstrated extensive variations in the effectiveness of mechanical circulatory assistance. This variation causes doubt to be cast on the simple-pump model. More extensive circulatory systems analyses to evaluate and optimize the control of mechanical assist devices are presented in Section 5.1 (Welkowitz et al. 1972; McMahon 1969). These more involved models still are not completely successful in explaining the clinical and experimental results obtained in many laboratories. For example, static models do not explain the stabilization of physiological parameters that often occurs after discontinuation of cardiac assistance (Hood et al. 1971). In addition, such models do not explain the differences in effect in assisting an animal with a normal heart as contrasted with assisting an animal with a failing heart (Feola, Halderer, and Kennedy 1971). In the latter case, the effect of the mechanical assistance is much greater than in the former. In order to explain some of these results, it can be demonstrated that the physiological control mechanisms must play a vital part in the effectiveness of mechanical left ventricular assistance (Welkowitz, Min, and Fich 1973).

A number of physiological studies have been carried out to demonstrate the involvement of the physiological control systems with the pumping process. These include:

1. studying the effects of therapeutic pumping on calculated muscle parameters
2. investigating the effects of therapeutic pumping on left ventricular power output and on power output divided by calculated maximum isovolumic stress in the heart muscle wall
3. measuring the effects of therapeutic pumping on cardiac output before and after pharmacological nerve block
4. measuring the effects of therapeutic pumping on peripheral resistance before and after pharmacological nerve block

5.3.1 Hemodynamic Parameters

A number of parameters have been explored in assessing the role of cardiac control mechanisms in assisted circulation. The ones that are discussed in this section include the spatially averaged maximum isovolumic wall stress of the left ventricle, the magnitude of the fundamental frequency ventricular diameter variation, left ventricular hemodynamic work and power, and aortic input resistance. Equation (5–14) defines the calculated spatially averaged maximum isovolumic wall stress in terms of the magnitudes of the source fundamental frequency phasors. From Eq. (2–22) one can derive the magnitude of the fundamental frequency ventricular diameter variation in terms of the same phasors as

$$L_m = K_L \frac{1}{\sqrt{Z_{gm}}} \qquad (5\text{–}33)$$

where K_L is a constant. Using the phasor components of the left ventricular pressure and aortic flow, the left ventricular hemodynamic power can be defined as

$$W_v = \sum_{n=0}^{\infty} P_{vn} Q_{an} \cos \theta_n \qquad (5\text{–}34)$$

where P_{vn} = Fourier series components of left ventricular pressure
Q_n = Fourier series components of aortic flow
θ_n = phase angles between these components

In addition, a useful parameter that was discussed in the exploration of the efficacy of balloon pumping is the ratio W_v/σ_{av}. The *aortic input resistance* R_{ai} is defined as the ratio of mean aortic pressure to mean aortic flow.

5.3.2 *Experimental Procedure*

A series of expeiments was carried out to demonstrate the involvement of the control system with the effectiveness of mechanically assisted circulation. These experiments were carried out on dogs under normal conditions, under induced heart failure, under failure with subsequent balloon pumping, and under all these conditions with pharmacological blockage of some of the neural control systems. They were performed on mongrel dogs weighing between 25 and 32 kg. The dogs were anesthetized with sodium pentobarbitol (25 mg/kg) and were maintained on artificial respiration. A left thoracotomy was performed. Left ventricular and aortic pressures were measured using polyethylene catheters placed in the left ventricle through the apex and in the root of the aorta through the left carotid artery. The catheters were filled with saline and connected to external pressure transducers. The aortic flow was measured using an electromagnetic flowmeter with the flow probe placed around the root of the aorta. For the experiments involving mechanical assistance, an intra-aortic balloon pump was inserted into the descending thoracic aorta through the femoral artery.

Failure of the left ventricle of the dogs was produced by ligation of all the branches of the left anterior descending coronary artery and a part of the circumflex artery. An animal was considered to be in failure when (1) cardiac output decreased by 30 percent or more or (2) the systolic blood pressure was reduced by 30 percent or more or (3) the left ventricular end diastolic pressure was increased to 12 mm Hg or more.

Pharmacological nerve block for both the sympathetic and parasympathetic nervous systems was produced using Atropine (3 mg/kg) and Inderal (0.5 mg/kg) injected intravenously. Atropine was injected very slowly for 5 minutes to block the parasympathetic system and Inderal for 3 minutes to block the sympathetic system.

5.3.3 *Results and Calculations*

As suggested, three different experimental and calculation techniques can be utilized to support the concept that the physiological control systems play an important role in establishing the effectiveness of mechanically assisted circulation. The combined weight of these different approaches appears quite convincing.

Effects of Induced Heart Failure and Mechanical Assistance on Calculated Muscle Parameters As indicated in Chapter 2, by appropriately using a balloon pump as a load on the left ventricle it is possible to calculate P_{gm} and Z_{gm} for normal and heart failure conditions. Using Eqs. (5–14) and

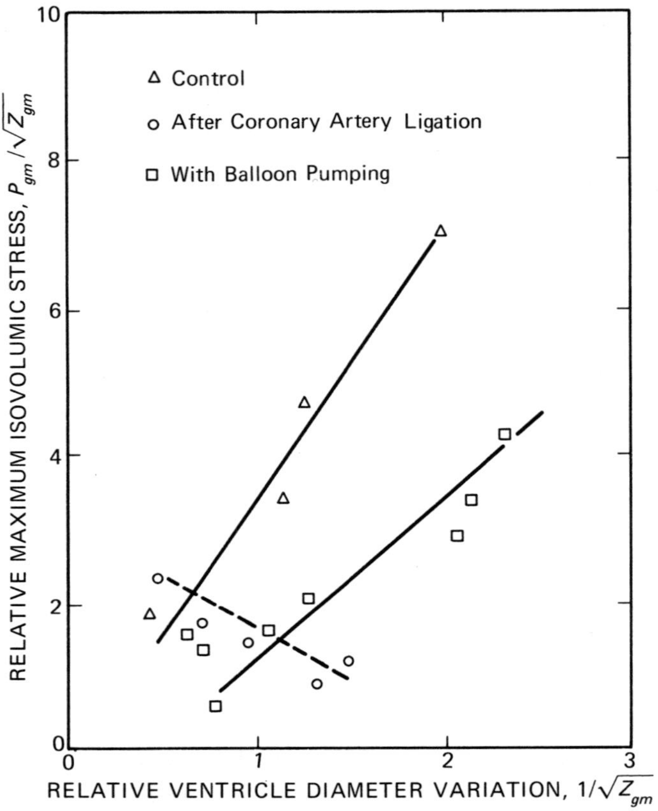

Figure 5–19 Calculated Peak Isovolumic Stress versus Diameter Variation before and after Induced Heart Failure and Subsequent Therapeutic Pumping.

(5–33), it is then possible to calculate the maximum isovolumic stress σ_{av} and the ventricular diameter variation L_m for the same conditions. A plot of calculated σ_{av} versus L_m was found to be a sensitive determiner of the status of cardiac muscle (Fich et al. 1973). Figure 5–19 shows the calculated peak isovolumic stress-length variation relationship first during normal ventricular function, then after failure induced by coronary artery ligation, and finally after mechanical assistance. In all three situations the nerve control systems were intact. A confirmation of this experiment is demonstrated in Figure 5–20 carried out on another dog, in which the plots of σ_{av} versus L_m are shown for the postcoronary artery ligation situation and then after mechanical assistance. It is apparent from these two figures that inducing a ventricular infarct produces a drastic effect on this calculated muscle characteristic. Furthermore mechanical assistance with small quan-

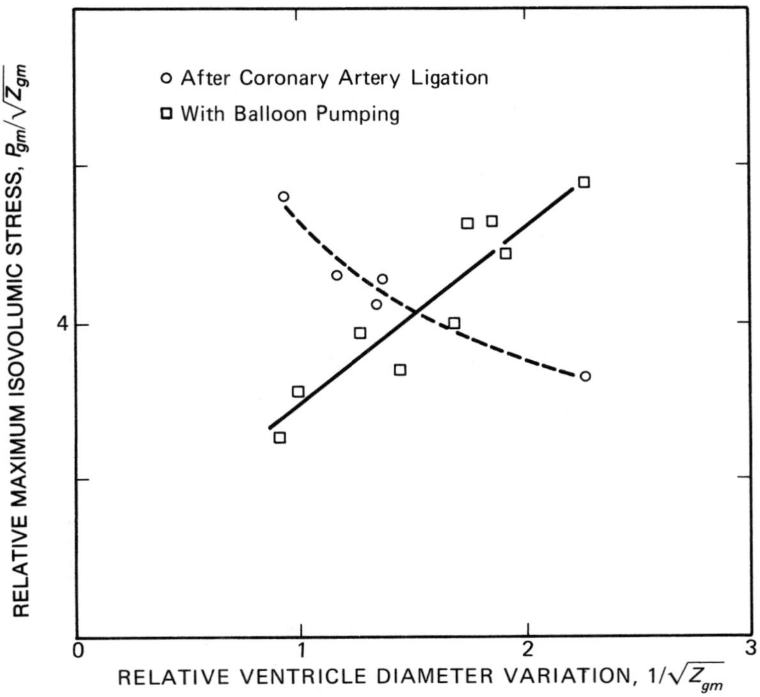

Figure 5–20 Calculated Peak Isovolumic Stress versus Diameter Variation after Induced Heart Failure and Subsequent Therapeutic Pumping.

tities of hydraulic energy produces an equally drastic recovery. A simple open-loop model of assistance as represented in Figure 5–5 cannot explain these results. It must be presumed that the intact neural control systems aid in the drastic change observed with mechanical assistance.

Effects of Therapeutic Pumping on Ventricular Hemodynamic Power and on the Pumping Figure of Merit (W_v/σ_{av}) It has often been proposed that a sensible determiner of cardiac state would be the ventricular hemodynamic power. Since the function of the heart is to pump blood through the circulatory system, a measure of its capabilities to perform this function appears to be a reasonable quantity to study. When a dog is in heart failure, it is not hemodynamically stable; thus it is not clear whether effective mechanical assistance should increase or decrease the ventricular hemodynamic power. This conjecture is supported by measurements in dogs in heart failure which showed that balloon pumping did not consistently

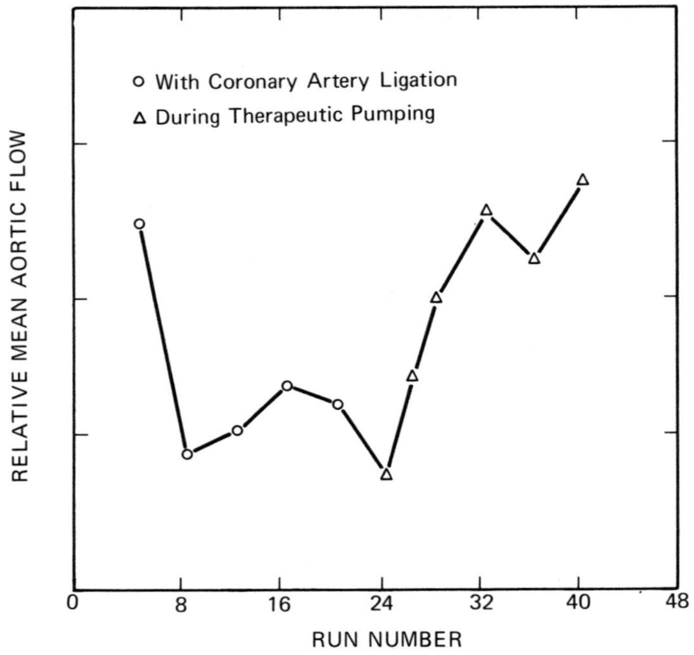

Figure 5–21 Measurements of Mean Aortic Flow during Heart Failure and Subsequent Therapeutic Pumping.

reduce the value of left ventricular power. However, as shown in Table 5–2, appropriately timed therapeutic pumping consistently decreased the ratio of calculated left ventricular hemodynamic power to calculated maximum isovolumic stress as defined by W_v/σ_{av} and computed from Eqs. (5–14) and (5–34) (Welkowitz, Min, and Fich 1973). The property of cardiac muscle represented by the peak isovolumic stress is under physiological control, and from the experimental results shown in Table 5–2 it appears to be a major factor involved in establishing the effectiveness of mechanical cardiac assistance. These results provide supporting evidence of the involvement of the physiological control systems in left ventricular in-series mechanical assistance.

Pharmacological Nerve Block The experimental results described thus far suggest that more direct evidence can be obtained to elucidate the role of the neural control systems. The most direct evidence results from the elimination of neural controls during circulatory assistance. Therefore, a series of experiments was carried out in which cardiac output (mean aortic

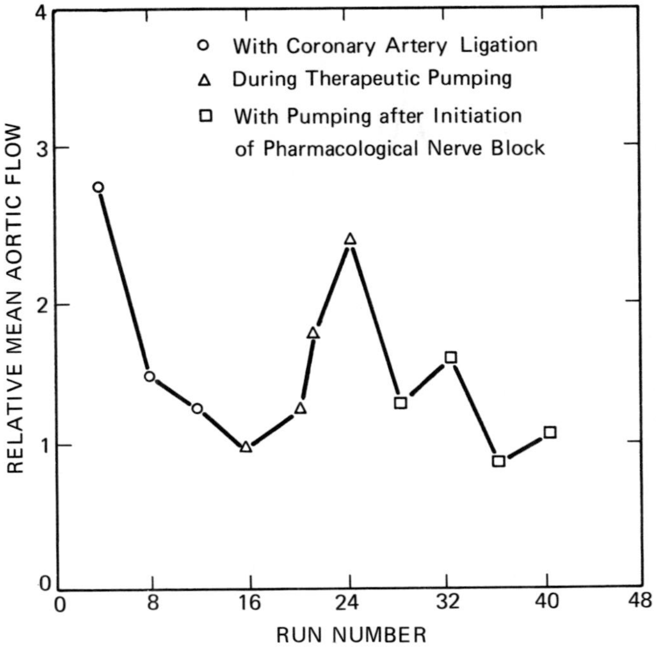

Figure 5–22 Measurements of Mean Aortic Flow during Heart Failure, Therapeutic Pumping, and Subsequent Pharmacological Nerve Block.

flow) and systemic resistance were measured for various conditions of heart failure and mechanical assistance both with and without pharmacological blockage of the neural controls. As indicated in the discussion of experimental procedures, both the sympathetic and parasympathetic nervous systems were blocked temporarily by using Atropine and Inderal.

Figure 5–21 demonstrates first the effect of heart failure induced by ligation of some branches of the coronary artery on the mean aortic flow, and then the effect of therapeutic pumping using a balloon pump. Figure 5–22 demonstrates the effect of heart failure, therapeutic pumping, and then pharmacological nerve block on mean aortic flow. It is apparent from a comparison of these figures that the stabilizing effects of mechanical assistance on cardiac output are eliminated when the neural controls are eliminated.

The results of the experiments in which aortic input resistance was studied are shown in Figures 5–23, 5–24, and 5–25. In the active experiments all, or a portion, of the following procedure was employed:

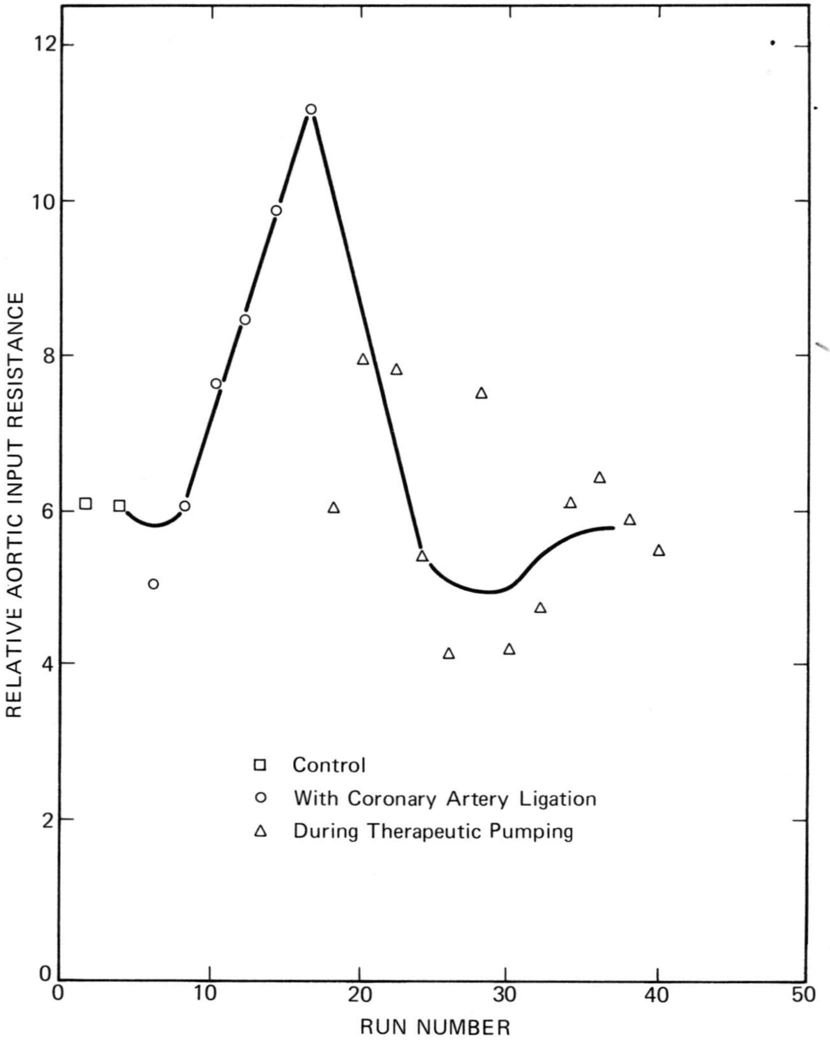

Figure 5–23 Measurements of Aortic Input Resistance during Heart Failure and Subsequent Therapeutic Pumping.

1. The initial input resistance of the aorta was measured.
2. After coronary artery ligation, the input resistance of the aorta was measured as the animal was going into failure.
3. When failure occurred, therapeutic pumping was initiated and the aortic resistance was measured during the pumping regime.
4. In the experiments in which the neural controls were eliminated, after

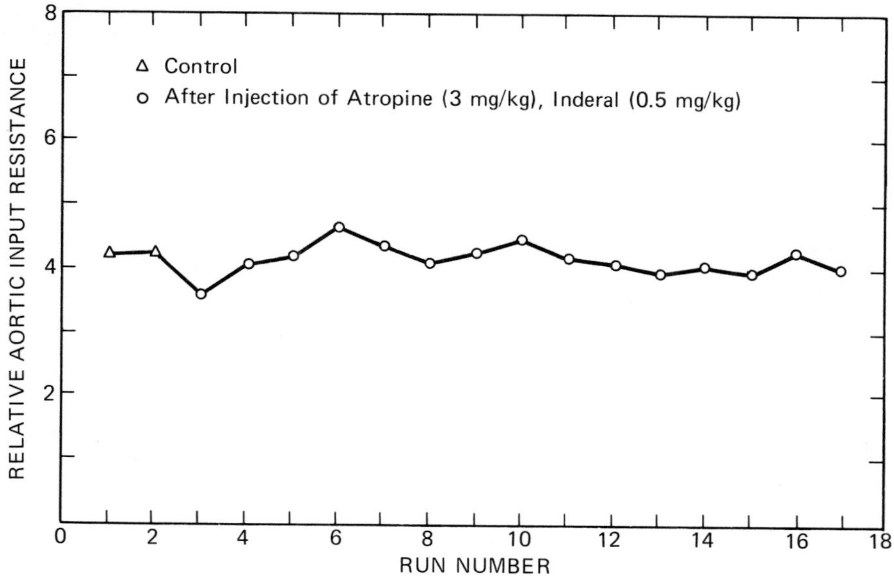

Figure 5–24 Measurements of Aortic Input Resistance before and after Injection of Atropine and Inderal.

a period of pumping when the aortic resistance had returned to approximately its initial value, pharmacological nerve blockage was induced and again the aortic input resistance was measured.

It can be seen from Figures 5–23 and 5–25 that, with both mechanical assistance and a functioning control system, the deterioration of the peripheral resistance due to the induced heart failure is corrected. However, after nerve blockage this correction could not be sustained. The control experiments exemplified by Figure 5–24 suggest that the final change in aortic resistance is not due to the effect of Atropine and Inderal.

5.4 Discussion of Results

The simple picture of mechanical assistance as a work reduction procedure is not sufficient to explain the efficacy of the technique and the stabilization of the improvements. The effect of the neural control systems also must come into play to produce satisfactory mechanically assisted circulation.

It would appear, from the results described, that the effect of left ventricular mechanical in-series assistance is to establish a cardiac state

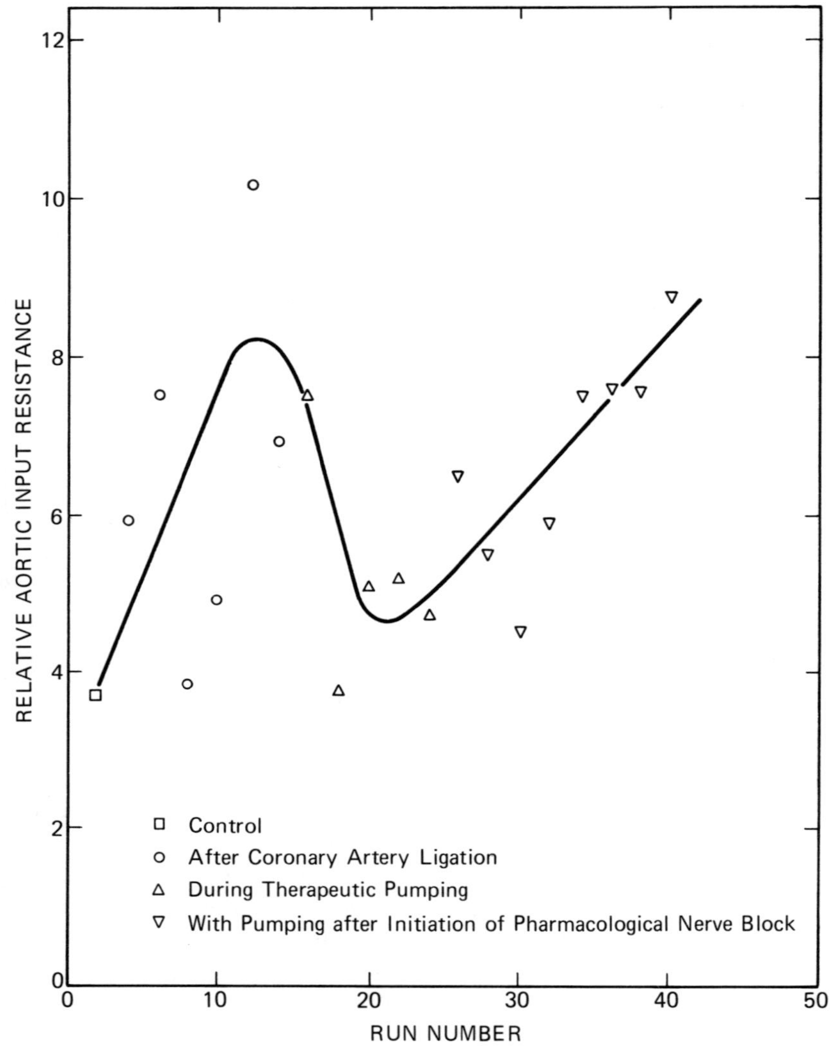

Figure 5–25 Measurements of Aortic Input Resistance during Heart Failure, Therapeutic Pumping, and Subsequent Pharmacological Nerve Block.

which permits the cardiovascular control system to produce almost normal blood flow throughout the body. The mechanical assistance permits this regulation even with a heavily impaired left ventricle. This necessary interaction of mechanical assistance with the physiological control system becomes more apparent when it is realized that in an in-series system (such as an intra-aortic balloon pump) the normal blood flow, when it is established, must all flow through and be pumped by the impaired heart (Welkowitz, Min, and Fich 1973).

References

Bryson, Y., and Ho, Y., *Apppied Optimal Control*, Blaisdell, Waltham, Mass., 1971, pp. 43–47.

Clark, J., "On the Feasibility of Closed-Loop Control of Intraaortic Balloon Pumping," *IEEE Trans. Biomed. Eng.* BME-30 (1973): 404–12.

Cooper, T., and Dempsey, P.J., "Assisted Circulation," *Mod. Concepts Cardiasc. Dis.* 37 (1968): 95 and 37 (1968): 101.

Feola, M.; Halderer, O.; and Kennedy, J.H., "Intraaortic Balloon Pumping at Different Levels of Experimental Acute Left Ventricular Failure," *Chest* 59 (1971): 68.

Fich, S.; Min, B.; Welkowitz, W.; Jaron, D.; and Kantrowitz, A., "Determination of Cardiac State," *Bibl. Cardiol.* 32 (1973): 72.

Fletcher, R., and Reeves, C.M., "Function Minimization by Conjugate Gradients," *Br. Computer J.* 7 (1964): 149–54.

Fox, R.L., *Optimization Methods for Engineering Design*, Addison-Wesley, Reading, Mass., 1971, pp. 52–55.

Goldfarb, D., "Mechanical Circulatory Assistance in the Treatment of Cardiac Failure," *Progr. Cardiovasc. Dis.* 12 (1969): 221.

Hood, W.D.; Joison, J.; Jumar, R.; Norman, J.; Hyberg, F.; and Urschel, G., "Experimental Myocardial Infarction, Effects of Intraaortic Balloon Pump Counterpulsation on Cardiac Performance in Intact Conscious Dogs with Left Ventricular Failure due to Coronary Insufficiency," *Cardiovasc. Res.* 5 (1971): 103.

Jaron, D.; Tomecek, J.; Freed, P.; Welkowitz, W.; Fich, S.; and Kantrowitz, A., "Measurement of Ventricular Load Phase Angle as an Operating Criterion for In-Series Assist Devices. Hemodynamic Studies Utilizing Intra-aortic Balloon Pumping," *Trans. ASAIO* 16 (1970): 466–71.

Kantrowitz, A., "An Intracorporeal Auxiliary Ventricle," in S.N. Levine (ed.), *Advances in Biomedical Engineering and Medical Physics*, John Wiley & Sons, New York, 1967, pp. 77–117.

———; Tjonneland, S.; Freed, P.; Phillips, S.; Butner, A.; and Sherman, J., "Initial Clinical Experience with Intraaortic Balloon Pumping in Cardiogenic Shock," *JAMA* 203 (1968): 113.

———; Krakauer, J.; Rubenfire, M.; Jaron, D.; Freed, P.; Welkowitz, W.; Cascade, P.; Wajsczuk, W.; Lipsius, M.; Ciborski, M.; Phillips, S.; and Hayden, M., "Initial Clinical Experience with a New Permanent Mechanical Auxiliary Ventricle: The Dynamic Aortic Patch," *Trans. ASAIO* 18 (1972): 159–67.

Kolff, W.J.; Moulopoulos, S.C.; Kwan-Gett, C.S.; and Kralios, A., "Mechanical Assistance to the Circulation: The Principle and the Methods," *Prog. Cardiovasc. Dis.* 12 (1969): 243.

Lee, T.; Adams, G.; and Gaines, W., *Computer Process Control, Modeling, and Optimization*, John Wiley & Sons, New York, 1971, pp. 215–17.

Liotta, D.; Crawford, E.; Cooley, D.; DeBakey, M.; deUrquin, M.; and Feldman, L., "Prolonged Partial Left Ventricular Bypass by Means of an Intrathoracic Pump Implanted in the Left Chest," *Trans. ASAIO* 8 (1962): 90.

McMahon, T.A., "The Dynamics and Fluid Mechanics of the Intraaortic Balloon Heart Assist Device," Ph.D. Thesis, M.I.T. Cambridge, Mass., 1969.

Min, B.G., "Analysis and Optimization of Cardiac Assistance by Intra-aortic Balloon Pumping," Ph.D. Thesis, Rutgers University, New Brunswick, N.J., 1972.

———; Welkowitz, W.; Fich, S.; Jaron, D.; and Kantrowitz, A., "Dynamic Optimization of In-Series Cardiac Assistance by Means of Intra-aortic Balloon Pumping," *Bull. Math. Biol.* 37 (1975): 19–35.

Moskowitz, M.S.; Freed, P.S.; Nachbar, J.G.; Von Recum, H.; and Kantrowitz, A., "A Self-Adjusting Intraaortic Balloon Pump Controller," *Proc. 29th ACEMB* (1976): 385.

Moułopolos, S.; Topaz, S.; and Kolff, W., "Diastolic Balloon Pumping in the Aorta—A Mechanical Assistance to the Circulation," *Am. Heart J.* 63 (1962): 669.

Shapiro, A.; Jaffrin, M.; Clark, C.; Murthy, V.; and McMahon, T., "Fluid Mechanics of Intra-aortic Balloon Counterpulsation," *Proc. Art. Heart Program Conf.* (1969): 505–14.

Shastri, S.J., "A Thevenin Equivalent Model of the Left Ventricle Derived from Hemodynamic Measurements Obtained by Use of a Ventricular Assist Pump," Ph.D. Thesis, Rutgers University, New Brunswick, N.J., 1969.

Welkowitz, W.; Fich, S.; Min, B.; Jaron, D.; and Kantrowitz, A., "Analysis of Assisted Circulation," *Bibl. Cardiol.* 29 (1972): 14–27.

———; Min, B.; and Fich, S., "The Interaction of Mechanical Left Ventricular Assistance and the Physiological Control System," in Iberall and Guyton (eds.), *Regulation and Control in Physiological Systems*, IFAC, 1973, p. 322.

Williams, M.J., Jr.; Welkowitz, W.; Fich, S.; Molony, D.A.; Jaron, D.; and Kantrowitz, A., "The Design of a Piezoelectric Heart Assist Device," *IEEE Trans. Biomed. Eng.* BME-22 (1975): 40–47.

6 Conclusion

An extensive analytical description of the systemic circulation is presented in Chapters 2, 3, and 4. One question that naturally arises is whether this detailed mathematical model contributes much more to the understanding of cardiovascular physiology or to applications in cardiology than the traditional experimental and intuitive investigations and presentations. In this chapter some of the areas that demonstrate the applicability of these mathematical techniques in cardiological diagnosis and therapy are discused. These include the design of automatic controllers for assisted circulation, the establishment of simple indices for the evaluation of left ventricular status, and the determination of cardiac output from pressure wave (internal) or pulse wave (external) measurements.

6.1 Automatic Controllers for Assisted Circulation

Chapter 5 describes at great length the analytical models that can aid in setting the proper timing sequences for appropriate therapeutic application of mechanical assistance, in modifying the pumping regime during the course of treatment, and in determining a suitable termination point for mechanical assistance. Hardware controllers (these may include computers) which incorporate some of these analytical concepts are described by Martin, Jaron, and Karlson (1976) and Moskowitz et al. (1976). In particular, the device described by Martin is specifically designed to implement the after-load phase angle criterion (180° phase difference between the fundental components of aortic pressure and aortic flow at the aortic root) that is described in Chapter 5. The adjustment accuracy of this instrument is designed to be one degree in phase angle, and it incorporates safety features to deactivate the assist device when there is a premature ventricular contraction.

6.2 Indices of Left Ventricular Status

Chapter 2 includes an equivalent source representation of the left ventricle as a pressure source in series with a hydraulic impedance. Using these parameters, Min et al. (1976) have calculated a zero-load aortic flow and

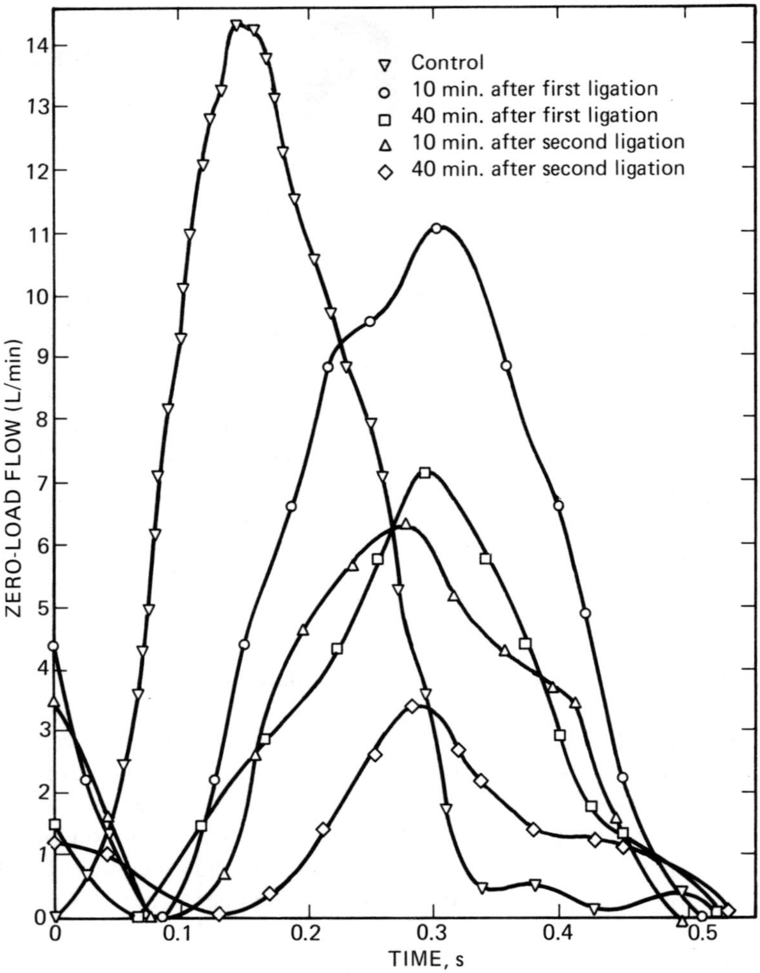

Figure 6–1 Computed Zero-Load Aortic Flow before and after Coronary Artery Ligation.

have demonstrated its utility as an index of severity of myocardial ischemia. Each phasor component of zero-load flow is computed from the corresponding phasors of source pressure and source impedance using the relationship

$$Q_s = \frac{P_g}{Z_g} \tag{6–1}$$

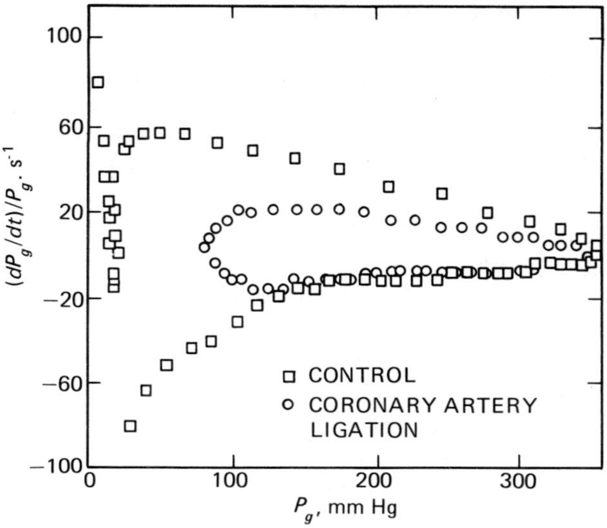

Figure 6–2 Computed Phase-plane Plot of P_g before and after Coronary Artery Ligation.

where Q_s is a phasor component of zero-load flow. Then the instantaneous zero-load flow waveform $Q_s(t)$ is computed by inverse Fourier analysis from the phasor components. The effect of successively increasing induced myocardial infarction on the computed zero-load flow is shown in Figure 6–1. While these changes in zero-load flow were occurring, only small changes took place in cardiac output, mean aortic pressure, and left ventricular pressure. Thus this computed index reflects the deterioration in ventricular function which is not reflected in the conventional parameters.

Using the same source parameters, Kresh et al. (1976) have shown that a phase-plane plot of $dP_g/dt/P_g$ versus P_g exhibits an inverse curvilinear relationship which is similar to that observed for $dP_v/dt/P_v$ versus P_v in experimental muscle mechanics preparations. As shown in Figure 6–2, in an animal with a myocardial infarction induced by ligation of branches of the left anterior descending coronary artery, the enclosed area diminishes greatly. These results indicate that this phase-plane plot may be a promising index of myocardial contractility and may prove more useful than other isovolumic indices (P_g is the isovolumic pressure that would exist in the left ventricle if the cardiac cycle were entirely isovolumic, rather than containing only a short real isovolumic phase).

6.3 Determination of Cardiac Output

The actual blood flow pumped by the left ventricle into the systemic circulation is obviously one of the most important measurements that can be made on the cardiovascular system. Totally invasive methods, such as the use of electromagnetic flowmeters placed around the aorta, are not suitable for most clinical applications. Thus many investigators have studied methods of obtaining blood flow from pressure measurements. These techniques are based upon various analytical representations of the vascular system, which simplify assumptions made to permit quantitative analysis. Most of these approaches have had limited accuracy—only approximations of the true flow waveform were obtained. Using the aorta model of Chapter 3 and improved optimization techniques, Muthukrishnan et al. (1975) carried out calculations of aortic geometry and flow from catheter measurements of pressure made on three dogs. The agreements between calculation and measurement of diameter and flow appear to be quite reasonable.

The extension of this method to noninvasive pulse contour measurements is presently being carried out. Two simultaneous pulse waves from above the carotid and abdominal arteries are measured using piezoresistive pulse transducers. Stroke volume is then calculated using the transfer characteristics of the aorta model of Chapter 3.

From these few examples, it appears that there are already useful applications of the analytical descriptions of the cardiovascular system presented in this book; hopefully in the near future many more such applications will be investigated.

References

Kresh, J.M.; Min, B.G.; Welkowitz, W.; and Kostis, J.B., "Computed Isovolumic Pressure Generating Capability of the Left Ventricle and a Related Myocardial Contractility Index," *Proc. 4th New England Bioeng. Conf.*, 1976, pp. 181–84.

Martin, P.; Jaron, D.; and Karlson, K., "A Digital Afterload Phase Angle Controller for In-Series Cardiac Assist Devices," *Proc. 29th ACEMB*, 1976, p. 238.

Min, B.G.; Kresh, J.M.; Welkowitz, W.; Fich, S.; Kostis, J.B.; and Mackenzie, J.W., "Changes of Computed Zero-Load Aortic Flow in Myocardial Ischemia," *Proc. 29th ACEMB*, 1976, p. 211.

Moskowitz, M.S.; Freed, P.S.; Nochbar, J.G.; Von Recum, A.; and Kantrowitz, A., "A Self-Adjusting Intraaortic Balloon Pump Controller," *Proc. 29th ACEMB*, 1976, p. 385.

Muthukrishnan, S.; Jaron, D.; Cooper, G.N.; and Karlson, K.E., "Determination of Blood Flow from Pressure Measurements: Preliminary Results," *Proc. 3rd New England Bioeng. Conf.*, 1975, pp. 322–33.

Index

Index

About the Author

Walter Welkowitz is a professor of electrical engineering at Rutgers University and director of the graduate program in biomedical engineering. He is also an adjunct professor in the Department of Surgery of the Rutgers Medical School. His research interests include the analysis of the performance of the cardiovascular system and the design of devices for mechanical assistance to the failing heart. For this work he was elected a fellow of the IEEE in 1976. Dr. Welkowitz is also active in the design of biomedical instruments and has recently published a book in this field entitled *Biomedical Instruments: Theory and Design* with S. Deutsch.